SMART CHOICES
FOR SMART PEOPLE

Eating healthy is in! And calorie counting is an important part of eating right. With this slim, handy reference, you'll get the latest accurate information you need to make wise, healthful food choices—wherever you are. Jam-packed with calorie counts, pocket-sized for easy portability, here's the biggest little book you can buy, perfect for the big year . . . **2000!**

Want to indulge in a treat? Enjoy! And let Corinne T. Netzer help you plan a day . . . a week . . . of guilt-free dining delight. She'll give you the tools you need to take the guesswork out of planning family meals . . . catching a bite at a fast-food restaurant . . . preparing a holiday feast . . . or navigating the supermarket aisles. Remember, you are in control of every bite you choose—with the guide that helps you eat wisely and well, at home or on the road!

THE
CORINNE T. NETZER
CALORIE COUNTER
FOR THE YEAR
2000

Corinne T. Netzer

A Dell Book

Published by
Dell Publishing
a division of
Random House, Inc.
1540 Broadway
New York, New York 10036

Dell books may be purchased for business or promotional use or for
special sales. For information please write to: Special Markets
Department, Random House, Inc., 1540 Broadway, New York,
N.Y. 10036.

Dell® is a registered trademark of Random House, Inc. and the
colophon is a trademark of Random House, Inc.

ISBN: 0-440-23498-0

Printed in the United States of America

Published simultaneously in Canada

September 1999

10 9 8 7 6 5 4 3 2 1

OPM

Introduction

The Corinne T. Netzer Calorie Counter for the Year 2000 has been compiled with a twofold purpose: as an annual to keep you up-to-date with many of the changes made by the food industry, and to provide a handy, put-in-purse-or-pocket volume.

To keep this book concise yet comprehensive, I have grouped together listings of the same manufacturer whenever possible. Many brand-name yogurts, for example, are listed as "all fruit flavors." Therefore, instead of three pages filled with individual flavors of yogurt, all with identical calorie counts, I have been able to use the extra space for many other products. And for many basic foods and beverages (such as butter, oil, milk, and alcoholic beverages) I have used generic listings, rather than include the numerous brands with the same or similar caloric values.

Finally, in the process of updating this edition, it was necessary to eliminate many previous listings and brands to accommodate new products and different brands. If you do not find a specific brand-name food that was listed in a previous edition of this book, this does not necessarily mean that the food product is no longer available. Also, since food producers are constantly revising and improving products, the caloric counts of your favorite food may have changed even if the description of the product hasn't. Be sure to check for updated entries.

This book contains data from individual producers and manufacturers and from the United States government. It contains the most current information available as we go to press.

Good luck—and good eating.

C.T.N.

Abbreviations

approx.	approximately
cont.	container
diam.	diameter
fl.	fluid
lb.	pound
oz.	ounce
pkg.	package
pkt.	packet
tbsp.	tablespoon
tsp.	teaspoon
w/	with

Symbols

"	inch
<	less than
*	prepared according to basic package directions

THE
CORINNE T. NETZER
CALORIE COUNTER
FOR THE YEAR
2000

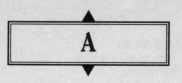

A

FOOD AND MEASURE   **CALORIES**

Abalone, meat only, raw, 4 oz. 119
Acerola, fresh, trimmed, ½ cup 16
Acorn squash, baked, cubed, ½ cup 57
Adzuki beans, boiled, ½ cup 147
Alfredo sauce, ¼ cup:
canned (Five Brothers) 110
canned *(Ragú)* 110
canned, w/mushrooms (Five Brothers) 80
refrigerated *(Di Giorno)* 230
refrigerated *(Di Giorno Light Varieties)* 170
refrigerated, mushroom *(Contadina)* 100
Almond, shelled:
(Beer Nuts Classic), 1 oz. 170
(Blue Diamond Smokehouse), 3 tbsp., 1.1 oz. 180
barbecue *(Blue Diamond),* 3 tbsp., 1.1 oz. 170
dry-roasted *(Arrowhead Mills),* ¼ cup 200
dry-roasted *(River Queen),* 1 oz. 160
honey-roasted *(Blue Diamond),* 3 tbsp., 1.1 oz. 170
hot and spicy *(Blue Diamond),* 3 tbsp., 1.1 oz. 190
natural, whole *(Blue Diamond),* 1.1 oz. 180
oil-roasted, salted, 1 oz. 176
roasted *(Blue Diamond),* 3 tbsp., 1.1 oz. 180
roasted *(River Queen),* 3 tbsp., 1 oz. 160
Almond butter *(Arrowhead Mills),* 2 tbsp. 210
Almond syrup *(Trader Vic's* Orgeat), 1 fl. oz. 100
Amaranth, boiled, drained, ½ cup 14
Amaranth, whole-grain, 1 oz. 106
Amaranth flour *(Arrowhead Mills),* ¼ cup 110
Amaranth seeds *(Arrowhead Mills),* ¼ cup 170
Anasazi beans, dry *(Arrowhead Mills),* ¼ cup 150
Anchovy, canned, in olive oil *(Duet),* 6 pieces 25
Angel-hair pasta:
dry, see "Pasta"

Angel-hair pasta *(cont.)*
refrigerated *(Contadina)*, 1¼ cups 230
refrigerated *(Di Giorno)*, 2 oz. 160
Angel-hair pasta entree, frozen *(Lean Cuisine)*, 10 oz. . 260
Angel-hair pasta mix, 1 cup*:
chicken broccoli *(Lipton* Pasta & Sauce) 260
Parmesan *(Lipton* Pasta & Sauce) 280
Anise seed, 1 tsp. 7
Apple:
fresh, w/peel, 2¾″ apple 81
fresh, peeled, 2¾″ apple 72
fresh, peeled, sliced, ½ cup 31
canned, diced, regular, or cinnamon flavor *(Del Monte*
Cup), 4 oz. 70
Apple, escalloped, frozen *(Stouffer's* Side Dish), ½ of
12-oz. pkg. 180
Apple butter, cider or spiced *(Smucker's)*, 1 tbsp. 45
Apple chips, all varieties *(Seneca)*, 1 oz. 140
Apple dip, 2 tbsp., except as noted:
candy or caramel *(Concord Farms)*, mix for 1 apple . . . 50
caramel *(Smucker's* Fat Free) 130
caramel *(T. Marzetti's)* 160
caramel *(T. Marzetti's* Fat Free) 110
peanut butter caramel *(T. Marzetti's)* 150
Apple drink blends, 8 fl. oz., except as noted:
berry burst *(Dole)* 120
berry pear *(Tropicana Twister)* 140
cranberry *(Tropicana)*, 11.5 fl. oz. 200
raspberry/blackberry *(Tropicana Twister)* 120
Apple juice, 8 fl. oz.:
(Hood) 120
(Minute Maid) 112
(Ocean Spray) 110
(Season's Best) 120
Applesauce, ½ cup, except as noted:
(Mott's) 100
(Mott's), 4-oz. cont. 90
(Seneca) 100
cinnamon *(Mott's)* 110
cinnamon *(Seneca)* 100

golden *(Leroux)*, 4-oz. cont. 80
golden delicious *(Seneca)* 90
McIntosh *(Seneca)* 100
unsweetened *(Mott's)* 50
unsweetened *(Seneca* 100% Natural) 60
Applesauce blends, 4 oz.
w/berry or cherry *(Leroux)* 80
w/mango and peach *(Fruitsations)* 70
w/mango *(Leroux)* 90
w/strawberry *(Fruitsations)* 90
Apricot:
fresh, 3 medium, 12 per lb. 51
fresh, pitted, halves, ½ cup 37
canned, halves *(Del Monte* Lite), ½ cup 60
canned, halves, in heavy syrup *(Del Monte)*, ½ cup . . . 100
dried, sulfured, 2 oz. 135
frozen, sweetened, ½ cup 119
Apricot nectar *(Libby's)*, 8 fl. oz. 150
Apricot syrup *(Smucker's)*, ¼ cup 210
Arby's, 1 serving:
breakfast items:
    bacon, 2 strips 90
    biscuit, plain 280
    croissant, plain 220
    danish, cinnamon nut 360
    egg portion 95
    french-*Toastix,* 6 pieces 430
    ham, 1.5 oz. 45
    sausage, 1.3 oz. 163
    Swiss cheese, .5 oz. 45
    table syrup, 1 oz. 100
roast beef sandwiches:
    Arby's melt w/cheddar 368
    Arby-Q 431
    bac'n cheddar deluxe 539
    beef'n cheddar 507
    Big Montana 686
    giant roast beef 555
    junior roast beef 324
    regular roast beef 388

Arby's, roast beef sandwiches (cont.)

super roast beef 523
chicken:
    breaded fillet 536
    Cordon Bleu 623
    chicken fingers, 2 pieces 290
    grilled BBQ 388
    grilled deluxe 430
    roast chicken club 546
    roast chicken deluxe 433
    roast chicken Santa Fe 463
sandwiches, sub roll:
    french dip 475
    hot ham 'n Swiss 500
    Italian sub 633
    Philly beef 'n Swiss 755
    roast beef sub 700
    triple cheese melt 720
    turkey sub 550
sandwiches, other:
    fish fillet 529
    ham'n cheese 359
    ham'n cheese melt 329
light menu:
    roast beef deluxe 296
    roast chicken deluxe 276
    roast turkey deluxe 260
    salad, garden 61
    salad, roast chicken 149
    side salad 23
potato, baked:
    plain 355
    w/margarine and sour cream 578
    broccoli'n cheddar 571
    deluxe 736
potato cakes, 2 pieces 204
fries:
    curly 300
    curly, cheddar 333
    homestyle, 2.5 oz. 212

homestyle, 4 oz. 340
homestyle, 5 oz. 423
soups, 8 oz.:
  Boston clam chowder 190
  cream of broccoli 160
  lumberjack mixed vegetable 90
  old fashion chicken noodle 80
  potato w/bacon 170
  timberline chili 220
  Wisconsin cheese 280
sauces/condiments:
  Arby's sauce, .5 oz. 15
  beef au jus, 2 oz. 10
  barbecue sauce, .5 oz. 30
  cheese sauce, cheddar, .75 oz. 35
  cheese sauce, Parmesan, .5 oz. 70
  horsey sauce, .5 oz. 60
  ketchup, .5 oz. 16
  mayonnaise, .5 oz. 110
  mayonnaise, light, .25 oz. 12
  mustard, .16 oz. 5
  sub sauce, Italian, .5 oz. 70
  tartar sauce, 1 oz. 140
dressings, .5 oz.:
  blue cheese 290
  buttermilk ranch, reduced cal 50
  honey French 280
  honey mayonnaise, reduced cal 70
  Italian, reduced cal 20
  red ranch 75
  Thousand Island 260
desserts/shakes:
  apple turnover 330
  cherry turnover 320
  cheesecake, plain 320
  chocolate chip cookie 125
  shake, chocolate, 12 oz. 451
  shake, jamocha, 12 oz. 384
  shake, vanilla, 12 oz. 360

Arby's, desserts/shakes *(cont.)*
   swirl, polar, 11.6 oz.:
      Butterfinger 457
      Heath 543
      Oreo 482
      peanut butter cup 517
      Snickers 511
Arrowroot *(Durkee),* ¼ tsp. 0
Arrowroot flour, 1 cup 457
Artichoke, globe:
fresh, boiled, 10.6-oz. choke 60
fresh, hearts, boiled, drained, ½ cup 42
canned or in jars *(Progresso),* 2.9-oz. piece 30
frozen, hearts, 9-oz. pkg. 96
Artichoke, Jerusalem, see "Jerusalem artichoke"
Artichoke appetizer, marinated:
(Progresso), 2 pieces, 1.1 oz. 50
Artichoke sauce *(Italia In Talola),* 2 tbsp. 110
Arugula, trimmed, 1 oz. 7
Asparagus, fresh:
raw, 4 spears, 3.8 oz. 14
boiled, 4 spears, ½″-diam. base 14
boiled, drained, cuts, ½ cup 22
Asparagus, canned, ½ cup, except as noted:
(Seneca) 20
all styles *(Del Monte)* 20
spears *(Green Giant),* 4.5 oz. 20
spears, extra large *(LeSueur),* 4.5 oz. 20
cuts *(Green Giant)* 20
Asparagus, frozen:
spears, boiled, 4 pieces 17
cuts *(Green Giant Harvest Fresh),* ⅔ cup 25
Asparagus bean, see "Winged bean"
Au jus gravy, canned *(Franco-American),* ¼ cup 10
Aubergine, see "Eggplant"
Avocado, California, 1 medium, 8 oz. 306
Avocado, cocktail *(Frieda's),* 1 piece, 1.4 oz. 60
Avocado dip *(Kraft),* 2 tbsp. 60

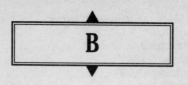

B

FOOD AND MEASURE   **CALORIES**

Babaganoush, see "Eggplant appetizer"
Bacon, cooked:
(Armour), 2 slices 60
(Oscar Mayer), 2 slices 60
(Oscar Mayer Center Cut), 2 slices 50
thick cut *(Oscar Mayer),* 1 slice, 1/8″ 60
turkey, see "Turkey bacon"
Bacon, Canadian *(Oscar Mayer),* 2 slices, 1.6 oz. 50
Bacon bits:
imitation, chips or bits *(Bac*Os),* 1½ tbsp. 30
real, bits or pieces *(Oscar Mayer),* 1 tbsp. 25
Bacon dip, 2 tbsp.:
horseradish *(Kraft)* 60
horseradish *(Kraft* Premium) 50
onion *(Kraft* Premium) 60
Bagel, 1 piece:
plain, mini *(Awrey's),* 9/10 oz. 100
plain or blueberry *(Awrey's),* 4 oz. 280
plain or cinnamon raisin *(Awrey's),* 2.6 oz. 200
plain, onion, or cinnamon raisin *(Wonder),* 3 oz. 210
blueberry or beefsteak rye *(Wonder),* 3 oz. 220
cinnamon raisin *(Awrey's),* 4 oz. 270
Bagel, frozen, 1 piece:
all varieties, except cinnamon raisin *(Sara Lee)* 210
plain or poppyseed *(Amy's)* 230
cinnamon raisin *(Sara Lee)* 220
cinnamon raisin or sesame *(Amy's)* 240
Baked beans, 1/2 cup:
(Allens) 150
(Campbell's New England Style/Old Fashioned) 180
(Friend's Original) 170
(Grandma Brown's Home Baked) 160
brown sugar and bacon-flavored *(Campbell's)* 170
w/bacon *(Grandma Brown's)* 150

Baked beans *(cont.)*
w/bacon and onion *(B&M)* 190
barbecue or honey *(B&M)* 170
honey *(Health Valley)* 110
w/pork *(B&M)* 180
w/pork *(Green Giant/Joan of Arc)* 120
w/pork *(Trappey's/Wagon Master)* 110
w/pork and tomato sauce *(Campbell's)* 130
w/pork and jalapeños *(Trappey's)* 130
red kidney *(B&M/Friend's)* 170
vegetarian *(B&M)* 170
yellow eye *(B&M)* 180
Baking mix (see also "Biscuit mix"), all-purpose:
(Arrowhead Mills), ¼ cup 140
(Bisquick), ⅓ cup 160
(Bisquick Reduced Fat)*, ⅓ cup 150
sweet *(Bisquick)*, ¼ cup 170
wheat free *(Arrowhead Mills)*, ¼ cup 120
Baking powder *(Calumet)*, ¼ tsp. 0
Balsam pear:
leafy-tips, boiled, drained, ½ cup 10
pods, boiled, drained, ½" pieces, ½ cup 12
Bamboo shoots:
fresh, raw, slices, ½ cup 21
fresh, boiled, drained, ½" slices, ½ cup 8
canned, drained, ½ cup 13
Banana, fresh:
(Frieda's Burro/Nino/Manzano/Red)*, 5 oz. 130
whole, 1 lb. 271
8¾" banana 105
red, 7¼" long 118
Banana, baking, see "Plantain"
Banana, dehydrated, ¼ cup 87
Barbecue glaze, Polynesian *(Trader Vic's)*, 2 tbsp. 45
Barbecue pocket, frozen *(Hot Pockets)*, 4.5 oz. 330
Barbecue sauce, 2 tbsp.:
(KC Masterpiece Bold/Original)* 60
(Kraft Char-Grill)* 60
(Kraft Original)* 40
(Kraft Extra Rich/*Kraft Thick'N Spicy* Original)* 50

garlic, hickory, hot, mesquite, or salsa style *(Kraft)* 40
hickory *(Kraft Thick'N Spicy)* 50
hickory, w/onion bits *(Kraft)* 50
hickory, mesquite, or spicy *(KC Masterpiece)* 60
honey *(Kraft)* 50
honey or mesquite *(Kraft Thick'N Spicy)* 60
honey Dijon *(KC Masterpiece)* 50
honey teriyaki *(KC Masterpiece)* 60
Italian seasonings or Kansas City style *(Kraft)* 45
Jamaican *(Helen's Tropical Exotics)* 60
Kansas City style *(Kraft Thick'N Spicy)* 60
onion bits *(Kraft)* 50
Oriental glaze *(World Harbors Cheriyaki)* 50
Polynesian *(Trader Vic's)* 30
teriyaki *(Kraft)* 60
tropical *(World Harbors Maui Mountain)* 50
Barley, pearled:
dry *(Arrowhead Mills)*, 1/4 cup 170
cooked, 1 cup 193
Barley flakes *(Arrowhead Mills)*, 1/3 cup 110
Barley flour *(Arrowhead Mills)*, 1/4 cup 93
Basil:
fresh, 1 oz. 8
fresh, 5 medium leaves or 2 tbsp. chopped 1
dried, ground, 1 tsp. 4
Bass (see also "Sea bass"), meat only, 4 oz.:
freshwater, raw. 129
freshwater, baked, broiled, or microwaved 166
striped, raw 110
striped, baked, broiled, or microwaved 141
Bay leaf, dried, crumbled, 1 tsp. 5
Bean dip, 2 tbsp.:
(Fritos/Fritos Hot) 40
black bean *(Old El Paso)* 25
black bean, spicy *(Valley of Mexico)*. 52
Bean dishes, see specific bean listings
Bean salad, canned or in jars, 1/2 cup:
three bean *(Green Giant)* 90
three bean *(Seneca)* 60
Bean sprouts, see "Sprouts" and specific listings

Beans, see specific listings
Beans, snap or string, see "Green bean"
Beans and rice, see "Rice dishes, mix"
Beechnuts, dried, shelled, 1 oz. 164
Beef, choice grade, meat only, trimmed to ¼" fat
  except as noted, 4 oz.:
brisket, whole, braised, lean w/fat 437
brisket, whole, braised, lean only 274
chuck, arm pot roast, braised, lean w/fat 395
chuck, arm pot roast, braised, lean only 255
chuck, blade roast, braised, lean w/fat 412
chuck, blade roast, braised, lean only 298
flank steak, trimmed to 0" fat, broiled, lean only 256
ground, broiled, medium, extra lean 290
ground, broiled, medium, lean 308
ground, broiled, medium, regular 328
porterhouse steak, broiled, lean w/fat 346
porterhouse steak, broiled, lean only 247
rib, whole, roasted, lean w/fat 426
rib, whole, roasted, lean only 276
rib, large end (ribs 6–9), roasted, lean w/fat 434
rib, large end (ribs 6–9), roasted, lean only 284
rib, small end (ribs 10–12), broiled, lean w/fat 376
rib, small end (ribs 10–12), broiled, lean only 264
round, bottom, braised, lean w/fat 322
round, bottom, braised, lean only 249
round, eye of, roasted, lean w/fat 273
round, eye of, roasted, lean only 198
round, full cut, broiled, lean w/fat 272
round, full cut, broiled, lean only 217
round, tip, roasted, lean w/fat 280
round, tip, roasted, lean only 213
round, top, broiled, lean w/fat 254
round, top, broiled, lean only 214
shank, crosscuts, braised, lean w/fat 298
shank, crosscuts, braised, lean only 228
short ribs, braised, lean w/fat 534
short ribs, braised, lean only 335
sirloin, top, broiled, lean w/fat 305
sirloin, top, broiled, lean only 229

T-bone steak, broiled, lean w/fat 338
T-bone steak, broiled, lean only 243
tenderloin, broiled, lean w/fat 345
tenderloin, broiled, lean only 252
top loin, broiled, lean w/fat 338
top loin, broiled, lean only 243
Beef, corned, see "Beef lunch meat"
Beef, dried, cured, 1 oz. 47
Beef, refrigerated, back ribs *(Lloyd's)*, 2 ribs w/sauce,
 5 oz. 360
"Beef," vegetarian (see also "Burger, vegetarian"):
canned *(Worthington Prime Stakes)*, 1 piece 120
canned *(Worthington Savory Slices)*, 3 slices 150
canned *(Worthington Vegetable Steaks)*, 2 pieces 80
canned, stew *(Worthington Country)*, 1 cup 210
frozen *(Worthington Meatless)*, 3/8" slice 110
frozen, corned *(Worthington Slices)*, 4 slices 140
frozen, smoked *(Worthington Slices)*, 6 slices 120
Beef dinner, frozen, 1 pkg.:
broccoli, Beijing *(Healthy Choice)*, 12 oz. 300
chicken fried steak *(Banquet Extra Helping)*, 16 oz. . . . 820
mesquite w/barbecue sauce *(Healthy Choice)*, 11 oz. . . . 320
patty, charbroiled *(Healthy Choice)*, 11 oz. 310
and peppers, Cantonese *(Healthy Choice)*, 11.5 oz. 270
pot roast, Yankee *(Banquet Extra Helping)*, 14.5 oz. . . . 410
pot roast, Yankee *(Healthy Choice)*, 11 oz. 290
Salisbury steak *(Banquet Extra Helping)*, 16.5 oz. 780
Salisbury steak *(Healthy Choice)*, 11.5 oz. 330
tips *(Healthy Choice)*, 11.25 oz. 260
Stroganoff *(Healthy Choice)*, 11 oz. 310
Beef entree, frozen, 1 pkg., except as noted:
broccoli and *(Stouffer's Skillet Sensations)*, 1/2 of 25-oz.
 pkg. 310
cheddar *(Stouffer's Skillet Sensations)*, 1/2 of 25-oz. pkg. . 600
chipped, creamed *(Stouffer's)*, 1/2 cup 160
chunky, and tomatoes *(Stouffer's Homestyle)*, 10 oz. . . . 280
enchilada, see "Enchilada entree"
fajita *(Lean Cuisine Skillet Sensations)*, 1/2 of 24-oz. pkg. . 300
home style *(Stouffer's Skillet Sensations)*, 1/2 of 25-oz.
 pkg. 360

Beef entree *(cont.)*

macaroni, see "Macaroni entrees, frozen"

w/mushroom gravy *(Banquet* Family), 1 patty w/gravy . . . 230
w/noodles, gravy *(Banquet* Family), 1 cup 150
w/onion gravy *(Banquet* Family), 1 patty w/gravy 180
Oriental *(Lean Cuisine Cafe Classics)*, 9¼ oz. 240
patty, grilled peppercorn *(Healthy Choice)*, 9 oz. 220
patty, w/vegetables *(Banquet* Meal), 9.5 oz. 310
patty, Western style *(Banquet)*, 9.5 oz. 380
pepper steak, green *(Stouffer's)*, 10.5 oz. 330
pepper steak, Oriental *(Healthy Choice)*, 9.5 oz. 250
peppercorn *(Lean Cuisine Cafe Classics)*, 8¾ oz. 220
pie *(Banquet)*, 7 oz. 400
pie *(Stouffer's)*, 10-oz. pie 440
pie, Yankee *(Marie Callender's)*, ½ of 16.5-oz. pie 640
pie, Yankee *(Marie Callender's)*, 9.5-oz. pie 560
portabello *(Lean Cuisine Cafe Classics)*, 9 oz. 220
pot roast *(Lean Cuisine American Favorites)*, 9 oz. 210
pot roast *(Marie Callender's)*, 1 cup 260
pot roast *(Stouffer's Hearty Portions)*, 16 oz. 370
pot roast, w/potatoes *(Stouffer's* Homestyle), 8⅞ oz. . . . 250
pot roast, Yankee *(Banquet* Meal), 9.4 oz. 230
roasted, oven *(Lean Cuisine American Favorites)*,
   9¼ oz. 260
roasted, w/potato *(Lean Cuisine Skillet Sensations)*,
   ½ of 24-oz. pkg. 290
Salisbury steak:
   (Banquet Meal), 9.5 oz. 380
   (Banquet Family), 1 patty w/gravy 230
   (Lean Cuisine American Favorites), 9½ oz. 280
   (Lean Cuisine Hearty Portions), 15½ oz. 340
   (Stouffer's Homestyle), 9⅝ oz. 380
   and macaroni and cheese *(Stouffer's)*, ⅙ of 68-oz.
      pkg. 420
   w/pasta shells *(Stouffer's Hearty Portions)*, 16 oz. . . . 570
   sirloin *(Marie Callender's)*, 14 oz. 550
sliced *(Banquet* Meal), 9 oz. 270
sliced, barbecue sauce and *(Stouffer's* Homestyle),
   10 oz. 370
sliced, w/gravy *(Banquet* Family), 2 slices w/gravy 100

steak, chicken-fried, w/gravy *(Marie Callender's),* 15 oz. . 650
steak, chicken-fried, w/mashed potato *(Marie Callender's
    Family Serve),* 1 patty, ½ cup pot. 600
steak, country-fried *(Stouffer's Hearty Portions),* 16 oz. . 560
steak, Philly *(Healthy Choice* Hearty Handfuls), 6.1 oz. . . . 290
stew *(Banquet* Family), 1 cup 160
Stroganoff *(Lean Cuisine Hearty Portions),* 14¼ oz. 350
Stroganoff *(Stouffer's),* 9¾ oz. 390
Stroganoff, w/noodles *(Marie Callender's),* 1 cup 600
teriyaki, and rice *(Lean Cuisine Skillet Sensations),* ½ of
    24-oz. pkg. 280
tips, Français *(Healthy Choice),* 9.5 oz. 280
tips, in mushroom sauce *(Marie Callender's),* 13.6 oz. . . . 430
tips, Southern *(Lean Cuisine American Favorites),*
    8¾ oz. 290
vegetables, country, and *(Lean Cuisine American
    Favorites),* 9 oz. 210
Beef gravy, canned, ¼ cup:
(Franco-American) 30
(Franco-American Slow Roasted) 25
(Franco-American/Franco-American Slow Roasted Fat
    Free) 20
Beef jerky, see "Sausage sticks"
Beef lunch meat (see also "Bologna," etc.), 2 oz.,
    except as noted:
cooked *(Boar's Head* Custom Cut No Salt) 90
corned *(Black Bear)* 60
corned *(Boar's Head* First Cut/Round) 80
corned *(Healthy Choice* Deli Zesty) 60
corned *(Healthy Deli)* 80
pepper, eye round *(Boar's Head)* 90
roast *(Healthy Deli)* 70
roast *(Oscar Mayer Deli-Thin),* 4 slices, 1.8 oz. 60
roast, Cajun *(Boar's Head)* 80
roast, Cajun *(Healthy Choice)* 60
roast, Italian style *(Healthy Choice)* 60
roast, Italian style *(Healthy Deli)* 70
roast, top round *(Boar's Head)* 90
top round *(Boar's Head* Cap-Off) 70
Beef pie, see "Beef entree, frozen"

Beef pocket, frozen:
and cheddar *(Hot Pockets),* 4.5 oz. 350
cheese steak *(Big Stuffs),* 5.4 oz. 440
cheese steak *(Deli Stuffs),* 4.5 oz. 350
Philly steak/cheese *(Croissant Pockets),* 4.5 oz. 350
Philly steak/cheese *(Lean Pockets),* 4.5 oz. 260
Philly steak/cheese melt *(Hot Pockets Toaster Breaks),*
    2.1 oz. 190
Beef sausage, see "Sausage"
Beef spread, roast beef *(Underwood),* ¼ cup, 2 oz. 140
Beefalo, meat only, roasted, 4 oz. 213
Beer, 12 fl. oz.:
regular 146
light 100
Beet, fresh:
raw, trimmed, sliced, ½ cup 29
boiled, drained, 2 medium, 2″ diam. 44
boiled, drained, sliced, ½ cup 38
Beet, canned, ½ cup, except as noted:
whole, baby *(LeSueur)* 35
whole or sliced *(Del Monte)* 35
whole or sliced *(Green Giant/Green Giant* No Salt) 35
whole or sliced *(Seneca)* 35
whole or sliced *(Seneca* No Salt) 40
Harvard *(Green Giant)* 60
Harvard *(Seneca)* 90
pickled *(Seneca),* 1 oz. 15
pickled, crinkle *(Del Monte)* 80
Beet greens, ½ cup:
raw, 1″ pieces 4
boiled, drained, 1″ pieces 20
Berliner, pork and beef, 1 oz. 65
Berries, mixed, frozen *(Cascadian Farm Harvest*
    Berries), 1 cup 65
Berry drink blend, 8 fl. oz.:
(Tropicana) 130
(V8 Splash) 110
Biryani paste *(Patak's),* 2 tbsp. 160
Biscuit, 1 piece:
(Awrey's Country), 2 oz. 140

(Awrey's Round), 1 oz. 70
(Awrey's Round), 2 oz. 150
(Awrey's Round Sliced), 3 oz. 230
Biscuit, refrigerated, 1 piece, except as noted:
(Big Country Butter Tastin') 100
(Grands! Extra Rich) 220
(Grands! HomeStyle) 210
(Grands! Butter Tastin') 200
(Pillsbury Country), 3 pieces 150
blueberry *(Grands!)* 210
buttermilk *(Big Country)* 100
buttermilk *(1869* Brand) 100
buttermilk *(Grands!)* 200
buttermilk *(Grands!* Reduced Fat) 190
buttermilk *(Pillsbury),* 3 pieces 150
buttermilk *(Pillsbury* Tender Layer), 3 pieces 160
buttermilk, flaky *(Hungry Jack)* 100
cinnamon and sugar *(Hungry Jack)* 110
corn, golden *(Grands!)* 210
flaky *(Grands!)* 200
flaky *(Hungry Jack)* 100
flaky *(Hungry Jack Butter Tastin')* 100
Southern style *(Big Country)* 100
Southern style *(Grands!)* 200
wheat *(Grands!)* 200
Biscuit mix, dry:
(Arrowhead Mills), 1/4 cup 120
(Gladiola), 1/3 cup 160
Black beans, dried:
(Frieda's), 1/3 cup, 3 oz. 120
boiled, 1/2 cup 113
turtle soup, dried *(Arrowhead Mills),* 1/4 cup 150
turtle soup, boiled, 1/2 cup 120
Black beans, canned (see also "Refried beans"),
    1/2 cup:
(Green Giant/Joan of Arc) 100
(Old El Paso) 110
(Progresso) 110
seasoned *(Allens/Trappey's)* 120
Black bean dip, see "Bean dip"

Black bean dishes, mix *(Fantastic Foods* International),
   ⅓ cup 160
Black bean sauce, 1 tbsp.:
(Ka•Me) 20
garlic *(Lee Kum Kee)* 25
Blackberry, ½ cup:
fresh, trimmed 37
canned *(Allens/Wolco)* 60
frozen *(Cascadian Farm),* 1 cup 80
Blackberry syrup
(Knott's Berry Farm), 1 fl. oz. 120
(Smucker's), ¼ cup 210
Black-eyed peas, ½ cup:
fresh or frozen, see "Cowpeas"
mature, dried *(Frieda's),* ⅓ cup, 3 oz. 130
mature, dried, boiled, ½ cup 100
Black-eyed peas, canned, ½ cup:
fresh shell *(Allens/East Texas Fair/Homefolks/Dorman)* . . 120
fresh shell, w/snaps *(Allens/East Texas Fair/Homefolks)* . 120
fresh, shell, w/jalapeño *(Homefolks)* 120
dry *(Allens/East Texas Fair)* 110
dry *(Green Giant/Joan of Arc)* 90
dry, w/bacon *(Allens/Sunshine)* 105
dry, w/bacon *(Trappey's)* 120
dry, w/jalapeño *(Trappey's)* 110
Blimpie:
6″ sub:
   Blimpie Best 410
   cheese trio 510
   club 450
   ham, salami, and provolone 590
   ham and Swiss 400
   roast beef 340
   tuna 570
   turkey 320
grilled chicken salad 350
Blood sausage, 1 oz. 107
Bloody Mary mixer:
regular or extra spicy *(Tabasco),* 1 cup 60
spicy *(Trader Vic's),* ½ cup 20

Blue squash, Australian *(Frieda's),* ¾ cup, 3 oz. 30
Blueberry:
fresh, ½ cup 41
frozen *(Cascadian Farm),* 1 cup 90
Blueberry, dried *(Frieda's),* ¼ cup, 1.4 oz. 140
Blueberry syrup:
(Knott's Berry Farm), 1 fl. oz. 120
(Smucker's), ¼ cup 210
(Smucker's Light), ¼ cup 130
Bluefish, meat only:
raw, 4 oz. 141
baked, broiled, or microwaved, 4 oz. 180
Boar, wild, meat only, roasted, 4 oz. 181
Bockwurst, raw, 1 oz. 87
Bok choy, see "Cabbage, Chinese"
Bologna (see also "Ham bologna," etc.):
(Black Bear German), 2 oz. 160
(Boar's Head), 2 oz. 150
(Diet Delight), 2 oz. 130
(Hansel 'n Gretel Classic/German), 2 oz. 150
(Healthy Choice Deli-Thin), 4 slices, 1.9 oz. 80
(Oscar Mayer), 1 oz. 90
(Oscar Mayer Free), 1 oz. 20
(Oscar Mayer Light), 1 oz. 60
beef *(Boar's Head),* 2 oz. 150
beef *(Diet Delight),* 2 oz. 150
beef *(Healthy Choice),* 1-oz. slice 35
beef *(Oscar Mayer),* 1 oz. 90
garlic *(Boar's Head),* 2 oz. 150
garlic *(Oscar Mayer),* 1.4-oz. slice 130
ring *(Oscar Mayer* Wisconsin), 2 oz. 180
"Bologna," vegetarian, frozen *(Worthington Bolono),*
   3 slices 80
Bonito, meat only, raw, 4 oz. 146
Borage, raw, 1″ pieces, ½ cup 9
Bouillon:
beef *(Maggi),* ½ tablet 15
beef *(Wyler's/Wyler's* Reduced Sodium), 1 tsp. 5
beef *(Wyler's/Steero* Very Low Sodium), 1 tsp. 10
beef or chicken *(Maggi),* 1 cube or 1 tsp. 5

Bouillon *(cont.)*
beef or chicken *(MBT/Wyler's)*, 1 pkt. 15
beef or chicken *(Wyler's/Wyler's* Reduced Sodium),
  1 tsp. 5
chicken *(Maggi* 2.5 oz.), ½ tablet 15
chicken *(Maggi* Dominican), ½ tablet 20
chicken *(Wyler's/Steero* Very Low Sodium), 1 tsp. 10
chicken and tomato *(Maggi)*, ½ tablet 15
chicken and tomato *(Maggi)*, 1 tsp. 5
onion *(MBT* Instant), 1 pkt. 15
vegetable *(Maggi* Vegetarian), 1 cube 5
vegetable *(MBT)*, 1 pkt. 10
vegetable *(Wyler's)*, 1 tsp. .5
Bow-tie pasta, see "Pasta, dry"
Bow-tie pasta dishes, mix:
chicken primavera *(Lipton* Pasta & Sauce), 1 cup* 290
w/creamy mushroom sauce *(DeBoles)*, 2.4 oz. 240
Italian cheese *(Lipton* Pasta & Sauce), 1 cup* 300
Bow-tie pasta entree, frozen, 1 pkg.:
Alfredo *(Marie Callender's)*, 13 oz. 620
and chicken *(Lean Cuisine Cafe Classics)*, 9½ oz. 250
and creamy tomato sauce *(Lean Cuisine)*, 10 oz. 260
marinara *(Marie Callender's)*, 13 oz. 430
and meat sauce *(Marie Callender's)*, 13 oz. 480
Boysenberry, fresh, see "Blackberry"
Boysenberry syrup:
(Knott's Berry Farm), 1 fl. oz. 120
(Smucker's), ¼ cup 210
Bran, see "Cereal" and specific grains
Bratwurst:
(Ball Park), 2-oz. link 190
(Boar's Head), 4-oz. link 300
(Hillshire Farm), 2.7-oz. link 230
Braunschweiger, 2 oz., except as noted:
(Black Bear Liverwurst) 180
(Boar's Head Lite Liverurst) 120
(Hansel 'n Gretel) 170
(Oscar Mayer), 1-oz. slice 100
spread *(Oscar Mayer)* 190
Brazil nuts, shelled, 1 oz., 6 large or 8 medium kernels . 186

Bread, 1 slice, except as noted:
bran, honey *(Pepperidge Farm)* 90
buttermilk *(Wonder)* 70
cinnamon raisin *(Wonder)* 70
French *(Wonder), 2″ slice* 140
hazelnut *(Monk's)* 70
Italian *(Wonder),* 2 slices 120
multigrain *(Wonder* Good Hearth/Fat Free) 70
oat bran or oat *(Roman Meal)* 70
oat bran and fiber *(Wonder)* 70
potato *(Arnold* Country) 100
potato *(Wonder/Wonder* Fat Free) 70
pumpernickel *(Wonder)* 80
pumpernickel, dark *(Pepperidge Farm)* 80
raisin *(Arnold Sun•Maid)* 70
raisin *(Monk's)* 80
rye *(Arnold* Deli/Real Jewish Dijon) 80
rye, Jewish *(Wonder)* 80
rye, soft *(Wonder Beefsteak)* 70
rye, soft, light *(Wonder Beefsteak),* 2 slices 80
sourdough *(Wonder)* 60
sourdough, light *(Wonder),* 2 slices 80
sunflower and bran *(Monk's)* 70
wheat *(Monk's* 100% Stoneground) 70
wheat *(Wonder* Split Top/Family) 70
wheat, honey *(Wonder)* 70
wheat, whole *(Wonder* 100%) 70
wheat, whole, soft or thin *(Pepperidge Farm)* 60
wheatberry, honey *(Arnold)* 70
white *(Arnold* Brick Oven) 80
white *(Arnold* Brick Oven 8 oz./1 lb.), 2 slices 110
white *(Monk's)* 70
white *(Pepperidge Farm)* 90
white *(Wonder),* 1.1-oz. slice 80
white *(Wonder* Texas Toast) 120
white *(Wonder/Wonder* Old Fashioned), .9-oz. slice 70
white, honey *(Wonder* Fat Free) 70
white or wheat *(Wonder Home Pride)* 80
white or wheat, light *(Wonder),* 2 slices 80
Bread, brown, canned, plain or raisin *(B&M),* ½″ slice . 130

Bread, refrigerated, French loaf, crusty *(Pillsbury),*
1/5 loaf 150
Bread mix (see also "Bread mix, sweet"):
cracked wheat *(Pillsbury* Bread Machine), 1/12 loaf* 130
Italian herb, honey oatmeal, or stoneground wheat
  (Fleischmann's Bread Machine), 1/3 cup, 1/8 loaf* 160
multigrain or rye *(Arrowhead Mills),* 1/3 cup mix 160
seitan *(Arrowhead Mills* Quick), 1/3 cup mix 160
sourdough *(Fleischmann's* Bread Machine), 1/3 cup,
  1/8 loaf* 150
spelt, whole wheat, or white *(Arrowhead Mills),* 1/3 cup
  mix 150
white, country *(Fleischmann's* Bread Machine), 1/3 cup,
  1/8 loaf* 170
white, crusty *(Pillsbury* Bread Machine), 1/12 loaf* 130
Bread mix*, sweet:
apple cinnamon *(Fleischmann's* Bread Machine), 1/8 loaf . 160
apple cinnamon *(Pillsbury),* 1/12 loaf 190
banana *(Betty Crocker* Quickbread), 1/11 loaf 180
banana *(Pillsbury),* 1/12 loaf 170
blueberry *(Pillsbury),* 1/12 loaf 160
carrot *(Pillsbury),* 1/16 loaf 140
cinnamon raisin *(Betty Crocker* Quickbread), 1/13 loaf . . . 190
cinnamon raisin *(Fleischmann's* Bread Machine), 1/8 loaf . 160
cinnamon swirl *(Pillsbury),* 1/12 loaf 220
corn bread, see "Corn bread"
cranberry *(Pillsbury),* 1/12 loaf 160
cranberry orange *(Fleischmann's* Bread Machine),
  1/8 loaf 150
date *(Pillsbury),* 1/12 loaf 180
lemon poppy seed *(Pillsbury),* 1/12 loaf 180
gingerbread *(Pillsbury),* 1/8 loaf 220
nut *(Pillsbury),* 1/12 loaf 170
pumpkin *(Pillsbury),* 1/12 loaf 170
Bread crumbs, 1/4 cup or 1 oz.:
plain or Italian *(Progresso)* 110
garlic-herb or Parmesan *(Progresso)* 100
Bread cubes, see "Stuffing"
Bread dough, see "Bread, refrigerated"

Breadfruit seeds:
boiled, shelled, 1 oz. 48
roasted, shelled, 1 oz. 59
Breadsticks:
plain *(Stella D'oro* Sodium Free), 1 pieces 45
plain or garlic *(Stella D'oro* Deli Style), 5 pieces 60
plain or garlic *(Stella D'oro* Grissini Style), 3 pieces 60
plain, garlic, or wheat *(Stella D'oro)*, 1 piece 40
buttery *(Awrey's Deli Stix)*, 2 pieces 130
dill and onion *(Awrey's Deli Stix)*, 2 pieces 130
garlic *(Stella D'oro* Fat Free), 2 pieces 70
garlic-pepper or Italian spice *(Awrey's Deli Stix)*,
    2 pieces 140
onion *(Stella D'oro)*, 1 piece 40
potato onion, cracked pepper, or salsa *(Stella D'oro)*,
    4 pieces 70
salted *(Stella D'oro)*, 4 pieces 70
sesame *(Stella D'oro)*, 1 piece 50
sesame *(Stella D'oro* Lowfat), 2 pieces 70
Breadsticks, refrigerated:
(Pillsbury), 1 piece 110
garlic and herb *(Pillsbury)*, 2 pieces 180
Breakfast dishes, see specific listings
Breakfast sandwich, frozen, vegetarian, 1 piece:
bagel *(Morningstar Farms Scramblers)* 320
English muffin *(Morningstar Farms Scramblers)* 240
English muffin, cheese *(Morningstar Farms Scramblers)* . 280
Breakfast syrup, see "Maple syrup" and "Pancake
    syrup"
Broad beans, boiled, drained, 4 oz. 64
Broad beans, mature:
dry, boiled, ½ cup 93
canned *(Progresso* Fava), ½ cup 110
Broccoli, fresh:
raw, 8.7-oz. stalk 42
raw, chopped, ½ cup 12
boiled, drained, 1 stalk, 6.3 oz. 51
boiled, drained, chopped, ½ cup 22
Broccoli, frozen:
(Seneca), 1 cup 25

Broccoli, frozen *(cont.)*
(Seneca Normandy/Stir Fry), 1 cup 30
spears *(Green Giant* Select), 3 oz. 25
spears, *(Green Giant Harvest Fresh)*, 3.5 oz. 25
spears, in butter sauce *(Green Giant)*, 4 oz. 50
florets *(Green Giant* Select), 1⅓ cups 25
florets *(Seabrook)*, 1 cup 25
cuts *(Green Giant/Green Giant Harvest Fresh)*, ⅔ cup 25
chopped *(Green Giant)*, ¾ cup 25
cuts *(Cascadian Farm)*, ½ cup 24
in cheese sauce *(Green Giant)*, ⅔ cup 70
in cheese sauce, cheddar *(Cascadian Farm)*, ½ cup 60
Broccoli combinations, frozen, ⅔ cup, except as noted:
w/carrots, cauliflower *(Green Giant* Select Skillet) 25
w/carrots, water chestnuts *(Green Giant* Select Stir-fry) . . 25
w/cauliflower:
   and carrots *(Green Giant Harvest Fresh)*, 1 cup 30
   and carrots, corn, sweet pepper, in butter sauce
    (Green Giant), ¾ cup 60
   and carrots, in cheese sauce *(Green Giant)* 80
and pasta, peas, corn, red pepper, in butter sauce
   (Green Giant), ¾ cup 70
Broccoli dishes, frozen:
au gratin *(Stouffer's)*, ½ cup 100
pot pie *(Amy's)*, 7.5 oz. 430
Broccoli rabe, fresh *(Frieda's* Rapini), ¾ cup, 3 oz. . . . 15
Broccoli-cheese croissant, frozen *(Sara Lee)*, 1 piece . . . 280
Broccoli-cheese pocket, frozen, 4.5-oz. piece:
(Amy's) 270
cheddar *(Ken & Robert's Veggie Pockets)* 250
Broth, see "Bouillon" and "Soup"
Broth concentrate, 2 tsp.:
beef *(Knorr)* 15
chicken *(Knorr)* 5
Brown gravy, ¼ cup, except as noted:
canned, w/onions *(Franco-American)* 25
mix* *(Pillsbury)* 15
Brownie, 1 piece, except as noted:
chocolate, Bavarian *(Awrey's)* 250
chocolate, decadent *(Awrey's)* 230

chocolate, peanut *(Awrey's* Sensation) 230
fudge *(Entenmann's),* ½ piece, 1½ oz. 200
fudge nut *(Awrey's)* 190
fudge nut, chewy *(Awrey's)* 210
fudge w/out nuts *(Awrey's)* 200
Brownie mix, 1 piece*:
(Arrowhead Mills) 110
(Arrowhead Mills Fat Free) 120
(Betty Crocker Original Supreme) 160
(Betty Crocker Pouch) 190
(Betty Crocker T-Rex Fossils) 180
(Betty Crocker Turtle) 170
caramel *(Betty Crocker* Supreme) 190
cheesecake swirl *(Pillsbury* Thick 'n Fudgy) 170
chocolate, dark, w/*Hershey's* syrup *(Betty Crocker*
    Supreme) 170
chocolate, double *(Pillsbury* Thick 'n Fudgy) 150
chocolate, German *(Betty Crocker* Supreme) 220
chocolate chunk *(Betty Crocker* Supreme) 180
chocolate chunk *(Pillsbury* Thick 'n Fudgy) 160
devil's food *(SnackWell's)* 140
fudge *(Betty Crocker* Supreme) 190
fudge *(Betty Crocker* Supreme Family) 170
fudge *(Pillsbury* 15 oz.) 150
fudge *(Pillsbury* 21.5 oz.) 190
fudge *(SnackWell's)* 150
fudge *(Sweet Rewards* Low Fat) 130
fudge *(Sweet Rewards* Reduced Fat) 140
fudge, chocolate, dark *(Betty Crocker* Supreme) 170
fudge, hot *(Betty Crocker* Supreme) 170
frosted *(Betty Crocker* Supreme) 210
peanut butter candy *(Betty Crocker* w/*Reese's Pieces)* . . . 180
walnut *(Betty Crocker* Supreme) 180
walnut *(Martha White)* 170
walnut *(Pillsbury* Thick 'n Fudgy) 190
wheat free *(Arrowhead Mills)* 120
Browning sauce:
(GravyMaster), ¼ tsp. 10
(Maggi), 1 tsp. 15

Brussels sprouts:
fresh, raw, ½ cup 19
fresh, boiled, .7-oz. sprout 8
fresh, boiled, drained, ½ cup 30
frozen, boiled, drained, ½ cup 33
frozen, baby, in butter sauce *(Green Giant)*, ⅔ cup 60
Buckwheat, whole-grain, ¼ cup 146
Buckwheat flour *(Arrowhead Mills)*, ¼ cup 100
Buckwheat groats:
brown *(Arrowhead Mills)*, ¼ cup 140
roasted, cooked, 1 cup 182
Buffalo wing, vegetarian, frozen *(Morningstar Farms)*,
　5 pieces 200
Buffalo wing sauce *(World Harbors* After Glow Hot
　Zings), 2 tbsp. 30
Bulgur (see also "Tabouli"):
dry *(Arrowhead Mills)*, ¼ cup 150
cooked, 1 cup 152
Bun, see "Roll"
Bun, sweet, 1 piece:
cheese *(Entenmann's)*, 3 oz. 300
cinnamon *(Entenmann's Light)* 160
cinnamon *(Krispy Kreme)* 220
sticky *(Entenmann's)*, 2.5 oz. 260
Bun, sweet, frozen or refrigerated, 1 piece:
apple cinnamon, iced *(Pillsbury)* 150
caramel *(Pillsbury)* 170
cinnamon *(Sara Lee)* 370
cinnamon, iced *(Pillsbury)* 150
cinnamon, iced *(Pillsbury* Reduced Fat) 140
cinnamon raisin, iced *(Pillsbury)* 170
orange, iced *(Pillsbury)* 170
Burbot, meat only:
raw, 4 oz. 102
baked, broiled, or microwaved, 4 oz. 130
Burdock root:
(Frieda's Gobo Root), ¾ cup, 3 oz. 60
raw, 7.3-oz. piece 112
boiled, 1″ pieces, ½ cup 55

Burger, vegetarian:
canned *(LaLoma Redi-Burger)*, ⅝″ slice 120
canned *(LaLoma Vege-Burger)*, ¼ cup 70
canned *(Worthington)*, ¼ cup 60
frozen, crumbles:
   (Green Giant Harvest Burger for Recipes), ⅔ cup 90
   (Morningstar Farms Recipe Crumbles), ⅔ cup 90
   (Natural Touch Crumbles), ½ cup 60
frozen patties, see "Burger patty, frozen"
mix, dry:
   (Fantastic Nature's Burger Original), ¼ cup or
     1 patty* 170
   (Worthington Granburger), 3 tbsp. 60
   barbecue *(Fantastic Nature's Burger)*, ⅓ cup or
     1 patty* 170
   chunks *(Loma Linda)*, ¼ cup 70
   granules *(Loma Linda)*, 3 tbsp. 70
   southwestern *(Natural Touch* Burger Kit), ¼ pkg. 90
refrigerated *(Morningstar Farms* Quarter Prime), 3.4 oz. . . 140
refrigerated garden vegetable *(Morningstar Farms)*,
   3.5 oz. 150
Burger patty, frozen, 2.5-oz. patty, except as noted:
(Fantastic Nature's Burger Classic) 110
(Fantastic Nature's Burger Original) 140
(Gardenburger Original) 130
(Gardenburger Veggie Medley) 100
(Green Giant Harvest Burger Original), 3.2-oz. patty 140
(Ken & Robert's Veggie Burger) 130
(Morningstar Farms Better'n Burger), 2.8 oz. 70
(Morningstar Farms Grillers), 2.25 oz. 140
(Morningstar Farms Hard Rock Cafe), 3 oz. 170
(Morningstar Farms Prime), 3.4 oz. 140
(Natural Touch Vegan Burger), 2.75 oz. 70
bean, zesty *(Gardenburger)* 120
black bean, Southwestern *(Fantastic Nature's Burger)* . . . 150
black bean, spicy *(Morningstar Farms)*, 2.75 oz. 110
black bean, spicy *(Natural Touch)*, 2.75 oz. 100
California or Chicago *(Amy's* Veggie Burger) 100
fire-roasted vegetable *(Gardenburger)* 120
garden grill *(Morningstar Farms)* 120

Burger patty, frozen *(cont.)*

garden vegetable *(Morningstar Farms)*, 2.4 oz.	100
garden vegetable *(Natural Touch)*, 2.75 oz.	110
Greek, classic *(Gardenburger)*	120
hamburger style *(Gardenburger* Fat Free)	100
hamburger style *(Gardenburger* Low Fat)	110
Italian *(Green Giant Harvest Burger)*, 3.2-oz. patty	140
mushroom, savory *(Gardenburger)*	120
roasted red pepper and garlic *(Fantastic Nature's Burger)*	130
Southwestern *(Green Giant Harvest Burger)*, 3.2-oz. patty	140
Texas *(Amy's* Veggie Burger)	130
tofu *(Natural Touch* Okara), 2.25 oz.	110

Burger King, 1 serving:

breakfast dishes:

biscuit	300
biscuit w/egg	380
biscuit w/sausage and egg	490
biscuit w/sausage, egg, and cheese	620
cini-minis, w/out vanilla icing, 4 rolls	440
Croissan'wich, w/sausage and cheese	450
Croissan'wich, w/sausage, egg, and cheese	530
french toast sticks, 5 pieces	440
hash browns, large	410
hash browns, small	240

breakfast components:

bacon, 3 pieces	40
ham	35
A.M. Express jam, grape or strawberry	30
vanilla icing, 1 oz.	110
whipped classic blend	65

sandwiches:

bacon cheeseburger	400
bacon double cheeseburger	620
Big King	640
BK Big Fish	720
BK Broiler chicken	530
BK Broiler chicken, w/out mayo	370
cheeseburger	360

chicken 710
chicken, w/out mayo 500
Chick'N Crisp 460
Chick'N Crisp, w/out mayo 360
double cheeseburger 580
Double Whopper 920
Double Whopper, w/out mayo 760
Double Whopper, w/cheese 1010
Double Whopper, w/cheese, w/out mayo 850
hamburger 320
Whopper 660
Whopper, w/out mayo 510
Whopper w/cheese 760
Whopper w/cheese, w/out mayo 600
Whopper Jr. 400
Whopper Jr., w/out mayo 320
Whopper Jr. w/cheese 450
Whopper Jr. w/cheese, w/out mayo 370
sandwich condiments:
  Bull's Eye barbecue sauce, ½ oz. 20
  ketchup, ½ oz. 15
  King sauce, ½ oz. 70
  tartar sauce, 1.5 oz. 260
Chicken Tenders:
  4 pieces 180
  5 pieces 230
  8 pieces 350
dipping sauces, 1 oz.:
  barbecue 35
  honey or honey mustard 90
  ranch 170
  sweet and sour 45
side orders:
  fries, small 250
  fries, medium 400
  fries, king size 590
  onion rings, medium 380
  onion rings, king size 600
dessert/shakes:
  Dutch apple pie 300

Burger King, dessert/shakes *(cont.)*
shake, chocolate, small 330
shake, chocolate, medium 440
shake, vanilla, small 330
shake, vanilla, medium 430
shake, syrup added, chocolate, small 390
shake, syrup added, chocolate, medium 570
shake, syrup added, strawberry, small 390
shake, syrup added, strawberry, medium 550
Burrito, frozen, 1 piece:
bean, black, vegetable *(Amy's)*, 6 oz. 320
bean and cheese *(Amy's)*, 6 oz. 280
bean and cheese *(Old El Paso)*, 5 oz. 300
bean and cheese *(Patio)*, 5 oz. 300
bean and rice *(Amy's)*, 6 oz. 250
beef and bean, hot, medium, or mild *(Old El Paso)*,
5 oz. 320
beef and bean, hot *(Patio)*, 5 oz. 320
beef and bean, medium *(Patio)*, 5 oz. 310
beef and bean, mild *(Patio)*, 5 oz. 330
chicken *(Patio)*, 5 oz. 290
pizza, cheese *(Old El Paso)*, 3.5 oz. 240
cheese, pepperoni *(Old El Paso)*, 3.5 oz. 260
cheese, sausage *(Old El Paso)*, 3.5 oz. 250
Burrito, breakfast, frozen *(Amy's)*, 6 oz. 230
Burrito dinner mix *(Old El Paso Kit)*, 1 piece* 290
Burrito seasoning mix:
(Lawry's), 1 tbsp. 30
(Old El Paso), 2 tsp. 20
Butter, salted or unsalted, 1 tbsp.:
regular *(Land O Lakes)* 100
whipped *(Land O Lakes)* 70
light *(Land O Lakes)* 50
light, whipped *(Land O Lakes)* 35
Butter, flavored:
honey *(Downey's)*, .5 oz. 60
honey *(Land O Lakes)*, 1 tbsp. 90
roasted garlic *(Land O Lakes)*, 1 tbsp. 100
Butter flavor sprinkles, plain or garlic-herb
(Molly McButter), 1 tsp. 5

Butter salt *(Durkee),* ½ tsp. 0
Butterbeans, see "Lima beans"
Butterbur, canned, chopped, ½ cup 2
Buttercup squash *(Frieda's),* ¾ cup, 3 oz. 30
Butterfish, meat only:
raw, 4 oz. 166
baked, broiled, or microwaved, 4 oz. 212
Buttermilk, see "Milk"
Butternut, dried, shelled, 1 oz. 174
Butternut squash:
fresh raw *(Frieda's),* ¾ cup, 3 oz. 40
fresh, baked, cubed, ½ cup 41
frozen, boiled, drained, mashed, ½ cup 47
Butterscotch baking chips, 1 tbsp.:
(Hershey's) 80
(Nestlé) 80
Butterscotch caramel topping *(Smucker's* Special
    Recipe), 2 tbsp. 130
Butterscotch syrup *(Smucker's* Sundae), 2 tbsp. 110
Butterscotch topping:
(Kraft), 2 tbsp. 130
(Smucker's Fat Free), 2 tbsp. 130

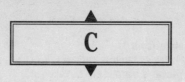

C

FOOD AND MEASURE	CALORIES

Cabbage:
raw, 5¾" head, 2½ lbs. 228
raw, shredded, ½ cup 9
boiled, drained, shredded, ½ cup 17
Cabbage, bok choy:
raw, shredded, ½ cup 5
boiled, drained, shredded, ½ cup 10
Cabbage, marinated, see "Kimchee"
Cabbage, mustard *(Frieda's)*, 1 cup, 3 oz. 20
Cabbage, napa *(Frieda's)*, 1 cup, 3 oz. 15
Cabbage, red or savoy, raw, shredded, ½ cup 10
Cabbage, stuffed, entree, frozen, w/whipped potato
    (Lean Cuisine), 9½ oz. 170
Cake:
almond-topped *(Entenmann's)*, ⅛ cake 180
apple crumb *(Entenmann's Orchard Delight)*, ⅛ cake . . . 260
banana loaf *(Entenmann's Light)*, ⅛ cake 140
banana chocolate chip *(Awrey's Marquise)*, 1/16 cake . . . 310
banana crunch *(Entenmann's)*, ⅛ cake 220
Black Forest torte *(Awrey's)*, 1/12 cake 350
blueberry crumb *(Entenmann's Orchard Delight)*,
    ⅛ cake 250
Boston cream *(Awrey's)*, 1/16 cake 190
butter *(Entenmann's Sunshine)*, ⅙ cake 310
carrot, iced, cream cheese *(Awrey's 2-Layer)*, 1/16 cake . 390
cheese coffee cake *(Entenmann's)*, ⅛ cake 160
cheesecake, pineapple *(Entenmann's)*, ⅕ cake 350
cherries cordial *(Awrey's Marquise)*, 1/16 cake 240
chocolate:
    chip crumb *(Entenmann's)*, ⅛ cake 370
    crunch *(Entenmann's)*, ⅑ cake 300
    double, buttercream *(Awrey's 3-Layer)*, 1/16 cake 310
    double, torte *(Awrey's)*, 1/12 cake 340
    German, buttercream *(Awrey's 3-Layer)*, 1/16 cake . . . 360

Cake, chocolate *(cont.)*

peanut *(Awrey's Marquise Fantasy)*, 1/16 cake 330
tropical *(Awrey's Marquise)*, 1/16 cake 230
white iced *(Awrey's 2-Layer)*, 1/16 cake 270
coffee cake *(Awrey's Long John)*, 1/12 cake 190
coconut, buttercream, yellow *(Awrey's 3-Layer)*,
1/16 cake 360
Danish ring cake *(Entenmann's)*, 1/5 cake 250
Danish twist cake, cheese *(Entenmann's)*, 1/8 cake 230
Danish twist cake, cinnamon apple or raspberry
(Entenmann's Light), 1/8 cake 140
Danish twist cake, lemon *(Entenmann's Light)*, 1/8 cake . . 130
espresso, French *(Awrey's Marquise)*, 1/16 cake 320
fruit *(Benson's Old Home)*, 4 slices, 4.6 oz. 470
golden, loaf *(Entenmann's Light)*, 1/8 cake 130
golden, fudge iced *(Entenmann's)*, 1/6 cake 340
lemon, buttercream *(Awrey's 3-Layer)*, 1/16 cake 320
lemon coconut *(Entenmann's)*, 1/6 cake 380
marble loaf *(Entenmann's Light)*, 1/8 cake 130
old-fashioned loaf *(Entenmann's)*, 1/8 cake 200
orange, buttercream *(Awrey's 3-Layer)*, 1/16 cake 330
peach or raspberry and cream *(Awrey's Marquise)*,
1/16 cake 260
pineapple loaf *(Entenmann's)*, 1/8 cake 220
pound, golden *(Awrey's)*, 1/6 cake 130
raisin loaf *(Entenmann's)*, 1/8 cake 220
raspberry nut *(Awrey's Marquise)*, 1/16 cake 310
rocky road *(Entenmann's)*, 1/8 cake 260
sour cream loaf *(Entenmann's)*, 1/8 cake 220
sponge, uniced, sheet *(Awrey's)*, 1/24 cake 190
strawberry *(Awrey's Supreme Marquise)*, 1/16 cake 240
strawberry torte *(Awrey's)*, 1/12 cake 270
yellow, white iced, sheet *(Awrey's)*, 1/24 cake 360

Cake, frozen:

Boston cream pie *(Mrs. Smith's)*, 1/8 pie 180
cappuccino *(Manzoni)*, 1/5 cake 220
cheesecake *(Sara Lee Original)*, 1/4 cake 350
cheesecake, cherry cream *(Sara Lee)*, 1/4 cake 350
cheesecake, chocolate mousse *(Sara Lee)*, 1/5 cake 400
cheesecake, French *(Sara Lee)*, 1/6 cake 350

cheesecake, strawberry cream *(Sara Lee)*, ¼ cake 330
chocolate, double, layer *(Sara Lee)*, ⅛ cake 260
chocolate, German, layer or coconut layer *(Sara Lee)*,
   ⅛ cake 280
coffee cake, butter streusel or raspberry *(Sara Lee)*,
   ⅙ cake 220
coffee cake, cheese *(Sara Lee Lowfat)*, ⅙ cake 180
coffee cake, crumb *(Sara Lee)*, ⅛ cake 220
coffee cake, pecan *(Sara Lee)*, ⅙ cake 230
fudge/golden layer *(Sara Lee)*, ⅛ cake 270
pound *(Sara Lee All Butter)*, ¼ cake 320
pound *(Sara Lee Lowfat)*, ¼ cake 280
pound, chocolate swirl *(Sara Lee)*, ¼ cake 330
pound, strawberry swirl *(Sara Lee)*, ¼ cake 290
strawberry shortcake *(Sara Lee)*, ⅛ cake 180
tiramisu *(Manzoni)*, ⅕ cake 230
vanilla layer *(Sara Lee)*, ⅛ cake 250
zabaglione *(Manzoni)*, ⅕ cake 240
Cake, mix, 1/12 cake*, except as noted:
angel food *(Pillsbury Moist Supreme)* 140
angel food, chocolate swirl or confetti *(SuperMoist)* 150
angel food, white *(SuperMoist One Step)* 140
banana *(Pillsbury Moist Supreme)* 250
butter pecan *(SuperMoist)* 240
butter recipe *(Pillsbury Moist Supreme)* 260
carrot *(Pillsbury Moist Supreme)* 250
carrot *(SuperMoist)*, 1/10 cake* 320
cheesecake *(Jell-O No Bake)*, ⅙ cake* 350
cheesecake, blueberry *(Jell-O No Bake)*, ⅙ cake* 320
cheesecake, cherry *(Jell-O No Bake)*, ⅙ cake* 330
cheesecake, strawberry *(Jell-O No Bake)*, ⅙ cake* 340
cherry chip *(SuperMoist)*, 1/10 cake* 290
chocolate *(Pillsbury Moist Supreme)* 250
chocolate, butter or chip *(SuperMoist)* 250
chocolate, butter recipe *(Pillsbury Moist Supreme)* 270
chocolate, dark *(Pillsbury Moist Supreme)* 250
chocolate, fudge, German, or double swirl *(SuperMoist)* . 270
chocolate, German *(Pillsbury Moist Supreme)* 230
chocolate, milk *(SuperMoist)* 240
chocolate caramel nut *(Pillsbury Bundt)*, 1/16 cake* 290

Cake, mix *(cont.)*
coffee cake, cinnamon *(Pillsbury* Streusel), 1/16 cake* . . . 260
coffee cake, chocolate chip *(Pillsbury* Streusel),
　1/16 cake* 270
devil's food *(Pillsbury Moist Supreme)* 270
devil's food *(SuperMoist)* 270
devil's food *(Sweet Rewards)* 200
fudge, marble *(SuperMoist),* 1/10 cake* 290
fudge, swirl *(Pillsbury Moist Supreme)* 250
Funfetti (Pillsbury Moist Supreme) 240
gingerbread *(Betty Crocker* Cake/Cookie Mix), 1/8 cake* . 230
lemon *(Pillsbury Moist Supreme),* 1/10 cake* 300
lemon *(SuperMoist)* 240
party swirl *(SuperMoist)* 250
peanut butter chocolate swirl *(SuperMoist)* 240
pineapple upside down *(Betty Crocker),* 1/6 cake* 400
pound *(Betty Crocker),* 1/8 cake* 260
rainbow chip or white sour cream *(SuperMoist),*
　1/10 cake* 280
spice *(SuperMoist)* 240
strawberry *(Pillsbury Moist Supreme)* 250
strawberry *(SuperMoist)* 250
strawberry cream cheese *(Pillsbury Bundt),* 1/16 cake* . 300
vanilla, French *(Pillsbury Moist Supreme)* 250
vanilla, French or golden *(SuperMoist)* 240
white *(Pillsbury Moist Supreme),* 1/10 cake* 270
white *(Sweet Rewards)* 190
white 'n fudge swirl *(Pillsbury Moist Supreme)* 250
white or yellow *(SuperMoist)* 250
yellow *(Pillsbury Moist Supreme)* 240
yellow *(Sweet Rewards)* 200
yellow, butter *(SuperMoist)* 260
Cake, snack (see also specific listings):
banana *(Tastykake* Creamies), 1.5-oz. piece 170
butter or marble *(Entenmann's),* 3-oz. piece 320
butterscotch iced *(Tastykake),* 2 cakes, 2 oz. 210
cheese puffs *(Entenmann's),* 3-oz. piece 330
cheese puffs, guava *(Entenmann's),* 2.8-oz. piece 290
chocolate *(Tastykake* Creamies), 1.5-oz. piece 180

chocolate, creme-filled *(Entenmann's Mini Cakes)*,
    2-oz. piece 220
crumb, French *(Entenmann's)*, 3-oz. piece 360
cupcake, butter cream or chocolate iced *(Tastykake)*,
    2 cakes, 2.25 oz. 250
cupcake, chocolate *(Tastykake)*, 2 pieces 220
cupcake, chocolate, creme-filled *(Entenmann's Light* Fat
    Free), 2-oz. piece 160
date-nut pastry *(Awrey's)*, 1.2-oz. piece 130
pound *(Awrey's)*, 2¼-oz. piece 210
vanilla *(Tastykake* Creamies), 1.5-oz. piece 190
Cake, snack, mix (see also "Brownie" and specific
    listings), 1 piece*, except as noted:
(Pillsbury M&M's) 170
(Pillsbury Oreo) 180
chocolate bar *(Betty Crocker Hershey)* 150
chocolate chip *(Pillsbury Chips Ahoy!)* 150
chocolate peanut butter bars *(Betty Crocker* Supreme) . 200
date bar *(Betty Crocker* Classic), 1/12 pkg. 150
dessert bar, easy layer *(Betty Crocker* Supreme) 140
lemon *(Sweet Rewards)*, ⅛ cake 170
lemon bar *(Betty Crocker Sunkist)* 140
lemon cheesecake *(Pillsbury)* 190
Calves' liver, see "Liver"
Cannelloni entree, cheese, frozen *(Lean Cuisine)*,
    9⅛-oz. pkg. 230
Candy:
almond, candy coated *(Blue Diamond* Jordan),
    13 pieces, 1.4 oz. 190
(Baby Ruth), 2.1-oz. bar 270
(Bittyfinger), 2 bars 170
(Buncha Crunch), 1.4-oz. bag 200
butter rum *(Pearson Nips)*, 2 pieces 60
(Butterfinger), 2.1-oz. bar 270
candy cane *(Spangler)*, 1 cane, ½ oz. 55
caramel, *(Kraft)*, 5 pieces 170
caramel, chocolate *(Kraft* Fudgies), 5 pieces 180
caramel, chocolate coated *(Rolo)*, 1.9-oz. pkg. 220
caramel and peanut butter *(Hershey's Sweet Escapes)*,
    1.4-oz. bar 150

Candy *(cont.)*

cherries, chocolate covered *(Perugina)*, 3 pieces 140
chocolate, assorted *(Godiva)*, 1.5 oz., approx. 3 pieces . . 210
chocolate, assorted *(Perugina)*, 3 pieces 170
chocolate, bittersweet *(Perugina)*, ½ bar 220
chocolate, bittersweet, w/hazelnuts *(Perugina Baci)*,
   3 pieces 250
chocolate, candy coated, 1.5 oz.:
   plain *(M&M's)* 210
   almond *(M&M's)* 230
   peanut or peanut butter *(M&M's)* 220
chocolate, dark:
   (Hershey's Special Dark), 1.45-oz. bar 230
   (Perugina), ½ bar 230
   w/almonds *(Ghirardelli)*, 1.5 oz. 220
   w/almonds or hazelnuts *(Perugina)*, ½ bar 240
   w/raspberries *(Ghirardelli)*, 1.5 oz. 210
chocolate, dark or milk *(Dove)*, 1.3-oz. bar 200
chocolate, milk:
   (Ghirardelli), 1.5 oz. 220
   (Hershey's), 1.55-oz. bar 230
   (Hershey's Hugs), 8 pieces 210
   (Hershey's Kisses), 8 pieces 210
   (Hershey's Nuggets), 4 pieces 210
   (Nestlé), 1.45-oz. bar 220
   (Perugina), ½ bar 230
   (Symphony), 1.5-oz. bar 230
   w/almonds *(Cadbury)*, 9 blocks 220
   w/almonds *(Ghirardelli)*, 1.5 oz. 230
   w/almonds *(Hershey's)*, 1.45-oz. bar 230
   w/almonds *(Hershey's* Golden), 2.8-oz. bar 450
   w/almonds *(Hershey's Hugs)*, 9 pieces 230
   w/almonds *(Hershey's Kisses)*, 8 pieces 210
   w/almonds *(Hershey's* Nuggets), 4 pieces 210
   w/almonds *(Perugina)*, ½ bar 240
   w/almonds and toffee *(Symphony)*, 1.5-oz. bar 240
   w/cappuccino filling *(Perugina)*, ⅓ bar 170
   w/caramel *(Caramello)*, 1.6-oz. bar 220
   cookies and cream *(Hershey's* Nuggets), 4 pieces . . . 200
   w/crisps *(Cadbury's Krisp)*, 9 blocks 200

w/crisps *(Nestlé Crunch)*, 1.55-oz. bar 230
w/crisps *(Ghirardelli)*, 1.25-oz. bar 180
w/crisps *(Krackel)*, 1.45-oz. bar 220
w/fruit, nuts *(Nestlé Chunky)*, 1.4-oz. bar 210
w/fruit, nuts *(Perugina)*, ½ bar 230
w/hazelnuts *(Perugina)*, ½ bar 240
w/macadamias *(Hershey's Golden)*, 2.4-oz. bar 380
w/macadamias *(Ghirardelli)*, 1.25-oz. bar 190
w/macadamias *(Perugina)*, ½ bar 240
w/peanuts *(Mr. Goodbar)*, 1.75-oz. bar 270
w/pecans *(Ghirardelli)*, 1.5 oz. 230
w/raspberry filling *(Perugina)*, ⅓ bar 150
w/toffee *(Ghirardelli)*, 1.5 oz. 220
w/toffee and almonds *(Hershey's* Nuggets), 4 pieces . 220
wafers *(Ghirardelli)*, 11 pieces 210
chocolate, mint *(Cadbury's* Mint), 5 blocks 190
chocolate, mint *(Ghirardelli)*, 1.5 oz. 220
chocolate, mint, cookies and *(Hershey's* Nuggets),
   4 pieces 200
chocolate, white *(Perugina)*, 1.5 oz. 250
chocolate, white, w/crisps *(Nestlé White Crunch)*,
   1.4-oz. bar 220
chocolate truffles *(Godiva)*, 1.5 oz., approx. 2 pieces . . . 220
coconut, w/chocolate *(Mounds)*, 1.9-oz. bar 250
coconut, w/chocolate and almonds *(Almond Joy)*,
   1.76-oz. bar 240
coffee *(Pearson Nips)*, 2 pieces 50
cookie bar, caramel *(Twix)*, 2 bars, 2 oz. 280
cookie bar, peanut butter *(Twix)*, 2 bars, 1.7 oz. 260
creme egg *(Milky Way)* 1.2-oz. egg 190
fruit chews, all flavors *(Starburst)*, 8 pieces 160
fruit flavor, all varieties *(Skittles)*, 1.5 oz. 170
fruit flavor, gummed, all flavors *(Amazin' Fruit)*, 1.9-oz.
   bag 180
gum, chewing, 1 stick:
   (Doublemint/Juicy Fruit/Big Red/Winterfresh/
     Wrigley's Spearmint) 10
   all varieties *(Freedent)* 10
   all varieties, sugar free *(Extra)* 5
hard, all flavors *(Hershey's Tastetations)*, 3 pieces 60

Candy *(cont.)*

hard, all flavors *(Jolly Rancher)*, 3 pieces 70
jelly beans *(Jolly Rancher Jolly Beans)*, 25 pieces 140
jelly beans *(Starburst)*, 1.5 oz. 150
licorice:
    (Nibs), 22 pieces 140
    (Pearson Nips), 2 pieces 60
    (Twizzlers), 4 pieces 140
    cherry *(Twizzlers)*, 4 pieces 150
    cherry *(Twizzlers* Pull 'n' Peel), 2.2-oz. pkg. 190
    chocolate *(Twizzlers)*, 5 pieces 140
    strawberry *(Twizzlers)*, 4 pieces 140
macadamia nuts:
    butter or coconut candy glazed *(Mauna Loa)*, 1 oz. . . . 190
    chocolate coated *(Mauna Loa)*, 4 pieces, 1.3 oz. 220
malted milk balls *(Whoppers)*, 1.75-oz. box 230
(Mars Almond), 1.8-oz. bar 240
marshmallow:
    (Kraft Funmallows), 4 pieces 110
    (Kraft Funmallows Miniature), ½ cup 100
    (Kraft Jet-Puffed), 5 pieces 110
    (Kraft Miniature/Cocoa Teddy Bear), ½ cup 100
    peanut *(Spangler)*, 6 pieces 163
(Milky Way), 2-oz. bar 270
(Milky Way Dark), 1.8-oz. bar 220
(Milky Way Light), 1.6-oz. bar 170
mint *(Kraft* Party), 7 pieces 60
mint, butter *(Kraft)*, 7 pieces 60
mint, chocolate coated *(York* Peppermint Pattie), 1.5-oz.
    bar 150
(Nestlé Turtles), 2 pieces 160
nonpareils *(Sno-Caps)*, 2.3-oz. box 300
(Nutrageous), 1.6-oz. bar 240
(Oh Henry!), .9-oz. bar 120
(100 Grand), 1.5-oz. bar 200
peanut, chocolate coated *(Goobers)*, 1.38-oz. bag 210
peanut brittle *(Kraft)*, 5 pieces 170
peanut butter, chocolate:
    (5th Avenue), 2-oz. bar 280
    candy coated *(Reese's Pieces)*, 1.6-oz. bag 230

cup *(Reese's)*, 1.6-oz. pkg. 240
cup *(Reese's* Crunchy), 1.6-oz. pkg. 250
peanut butter parfait *(Pearson Nips)*, 2 pieces 60
(Perugina After Eight), ⅓ bar 150
pretzel, milk or white chocolate coated *(Flipz)*, 1 oz. . . . 130
raisins, chocolate coated *(Raisinets)*, 1.58-oz. bag 200
(3 Musketeers), 2.1-oz. bar 260
toffee bar *(Heath)*, 1.4-oz. bar 210
toffee bar *(Skor)*, 1.4-oz. bar 220
toffee, bits *(Heath)*, ½ oz. 80
toffee, bits *(Heath Bits O' Brickle)*, ½ oz. 80
wafer, chocolate coated *(Kit Kat)*, 1.5-oz. bar 220
(Whatchamacallit), 1.7-oz. bar 250
Cane syrup, 1 tbsp. 52
Cannellini beans, see "Kidney beans"
Cannelloni dinner, frozen *(Amy's)*, 9 oz. 330
Cannelloni entree, cheese, frozen *(Lean Cuisine)*,
    9⅛ oz. 230
Cantaloupe, ½ of 5″ melon 94
Capers *(Crosse & Blackwell)*, 1 tbsp. 5
Capon, see "Chicken"
Cappicola, see "Ham lunch meat"
Cappuccino (see also "Coffee, flavored, mix"), iced,
    8 fl. oz.:
coffee *(Maxwell House Cappio)* 130
mocha or vanilla *(Maxwell House Cappio)* 140
Carambola, 1 medium, 4.7 oz. 42
Caramel custard, see "Pudding mix"
Caramel syrup *(Smucker's* Sundae), 2 tbsp. 110
Caramel topping, 2 tbsp.:
(Kraft) 120
(Smucker's Fat Free) 130
(Smucker's Microwave) 110
hot *(Smucker's)* 120
Caraway seeds, 1 tsp. 7
Cardamom, ground or seed, 1 tsp. 6
Carob drink mix, powder, 3 tsp. 45
Carp, meat only:
raw, 4 oz. 144
baked, broiled, or microwaved, 4 oz. 184

Carrot, fresh:
raw, whole, 7½″ long, 2.8 oz. 31
raw, whole, baby, 1 medium, 2¾″ long 4
raw, shredded, ½ cup 24
boiled, drained, sliced, ½ cup 35
Carrot, canned, ½ cup, sliced, except as noted:
(Del Monte) 35
(Green Giant) 25
(Seneca/Seneca No Salt) 25
baby, whole *(LeSueur)* 35
Carrot, frozen:
boiled, drained, sliced, ½ cup 26
baby *(Cascadian Farm),* 1 cup 60
baby, cut *(Green Giant),* ¾ cup 30
baby, cut *(Green Giant Harvest Fresh),* ⅔ cup 20
honey glazed *(Green Giant),* 1 cup 90
Carrot juice, canned, 8 fl. oz. 98
Cashew:
(Beer Nuts Classic), 1 oz. 170
(Frito-Lay), 1 oz. 180
(River Queen Fancy/Halves), ¼ cup, 1.2 oz. 190
(River Queen Fancy Unsalted), ¼ cup, 1.2 oz. 200
dry-roasted *(River Queen),* 1 oz. 160
dry-roasted, 1 oz. or 18 medium 163
honey-roasted *(River Queen* Halves), ¼ cup, 1.2 oz. 180
oil-roasted, 1 oz. or 18 medium 163
Cashew butter *(Arrowhead Mills),* 2 tbsp. 160
Catfish, channel, meat only:
farmed, raw, 4 oz. 153
farmed, baked, broiled, or microwaved, 4 oz. 172
wild, raw, 4 oz. 108
wild, baked, broiled, or microwaved, 4 oz. 119
Catjang, boiled, ½ cup 100
Catsup, see "Ketchup"
Cauliflower, fresh:
fresh, raw, 1″ pieces, ½ cup 13
fresh, raw, florets *(Dole),* 3 oz. 20
fresh, boiled, drained, 1″ pieces, ½ cup 14
fresh, green, raw, ⅕ head 28
frozen, florets *(Green Giant),* 1 cup 25

frozen, in cheese sauce *(Green Giant)*, ½ cup 60
Caviar (see also "Roe"), 1 tbsp.:
lumpfish, black or red *(Romanoff)* 15
salmon, red *(Romanoff)* 35
Caviar spread *(Krinos* Taramosalata), 1 tbsp. 90
Celeriac, fresh, raw, trimmed, ½ cup 31
Celery:
raw, 7½″-stalk, 1.6 oz. 6
raw, diced, ½ cup 10
boiled, drained, diced, ½ cup 13
Celery, Chinese *(Frieda's* Kun Choy), 1 cup, 3 oz. 15
Celery, dried, flakes or seed *(Tone's)*, 1 tsp. 9
Celery, frozen *(Seneca)*, ¾ cup 10
Celery root, see "Celeriac"
Celery salt *(Tone's)*, 1 tsp. 6
Cereal, ready-to-eat (see also specific grains):
all varieties *(Health Valley* Healthy Crunchies & Flakes),
   ¾ cup 130
amaranth flakes *(Arrowhead Mills)*, 1 cup 128
bran *(Multi-Bran Chex)*, 1 cup 200
bran *(Nabisco 100% Bran)*, ⅓ cup 80
bran *(Post Bran'nola)*, ½ cup 200
bran flakes *(Kellogg's All-Bran)*, ½ cup 80
bran flakes *(Post)*, ⅔ cup 90
bran w/raisins *(Kellogg's)*, 1 cup 200
bran w/raisins *(Post)*, 1 cup 190
bran w/raisins *(Post Bran'nola)*, ½ cup 200
buckwheat flakes, maple *(Arrowhead Mills)*, 1 cup 160
corn *(Corn Bursts)*, 1 cup 120
corn, blue bran flakes *(Health Valley)*, ¾ cup 100
corn, puffed, sweetened *(Kellogg's Corn Pops)*, 1 cup . . . 120
corn flakes *(Country)*, 1 cup 120
corn flakes *(Kellogg's)*, 1 cup 100
corn flakes *(Total)*, 1⅓ cups 110
corn flakes, w/ginseng *(New Morning)*, ¾ cup 110
corn and rice *(Kellogg's Crispix)*, 1 cup 110
flax, golden *(Health Valley)*, ½ cup 190
granola *(C.W. Post)*, ⅔ cup 280
granola *(Kellogg's* Lowfat), ½ cup 190

Cereal, ready-to-eat *(cont.)*

granola, all varieties *(Health Valley 98% Fat Free)*,
²/₃ cup 180
granola, w/fruit *(Nature Valley Lowfat)*, ²/₃ cup 210
granola, w/honey *(New Morning)*, ³/₄ cup 200
granola, w/raisins *(Heartland)*, ¹/₂ cup 290
granola, w/raisins *(Kellogg's Lowfat)*, ²/₃ cup 220
kamut flakes *(Arrowhead Mills)*, 1 cup 110
millet, puffed *(Arrowhead Mills)*, 1 cup 60
multigrain (see also "granola," above):
  (Basic 4), 1 cup 200
  (Cinnamon Grahams), ³/₄ cup 120
  (Cinnamon Toast Crunch), ³/₄ cup 130
  (Fiber One), ¹/₂ cup 60
  (French Toast Crunch), ³/₄ cup 120
  (Golden Crisp), ³/₄ cup 110
  (Golden Puffs), ³/₄ cup 100
  (Grape-Nuts), ¹/₂ cup 200
  (Grape-Nuts Flakes), ³/₄ cup 100
  (Honey Nut Chex), ³/₄ cup 120
  (Honey Nut Clusters) 1 cup 210
  (Honeycomb), 1¹/₃ cups 110
  (Kellogg's Apple Jacks/Fruit Loops), 1 cup 120
  (Kellogg's Healthy Choice Flakes), ³/₄ cup 110
  (Kellogg's Healthy Choice Squares), 1 cup 190
  (Kellogg's Just Right), 1 cup 210
  (Kellogg's Nutri-Grain), 1¹/₄ cups 180
  (Kellogg's Product 19), 1 cup 100
  (Kix), 1¹/₃ cups 120
  (Multi-Grain Cheerios Plus), 1 cup 110
  (Team Cheerios), 1 cup 120
  (Nabisco Team Flakes), 1¹/₄ cups 220
  (Total Whole Grain), ³/₄ cup 110
  (Trix), 1 cup 120
  w/almonds, raisins *(Kellogg's Healthy Choice)*, 1 cup . 210
  w/fruit, nuts *(Kellogg's Just Right)*, 1 cup 220
  w/fruit, nuts *(Kellogg's Mueslix)*, ³/₄ cup 200
  w/pecans *(Great Grains)*, ²/₃ cup 220
  raisins, dates, pecans *(Great Grains)*, ²/₃ cup 210

oat:
    (Arrowhead Mills Nature O's), 1 cup 130
    (Cheerios), 1 cup 110
    (Honey Bunches of Oats), ¾ cup 120
    (New Morning Oatios), 1 cup 120
    (Toasty O's), 1 cup 110
    w/almond *(Honey Bunches of Oats)*, ¾ cup . . . 130
    w/almond *(Oatmeal Crisp)*, 1 cup 220
    w/almond *(New Morning Oatios)*, 1 cup 100
    apple cinnamon *(Cheerios)*, ¾ cup 120
    w/blueberries *(New Morning Oatiola)*, 1 cup . . 200
    w/marshmallow *(Lucky Charms)*, 1 cup 120
    w/raisin *(Oatmeal Crisp)*, 1 cup 210
    sweetened *(Alpha-Bits)*, 1 cup 130
    sweetened *(Frosted Cheerios/Honey Nut Cheerios)*,
      1 cup 120
    sweetened *(Honey Nut Toasty O's)*, 1 cup 110
oat bran *(Health Valley* O's), ¾ cup 100
oat bran *(Kellogg's Cracklin' Oat Bran)*, ¾ cup 190
oat bran, apple cinnamon *(Health Valley 10 Bran O's)*,
    ¾ cup 100
oat bran, w/ginkgo *(New Morning GinkgO's)*, 1 cup 120
oat bran flakes *(Health Valley)*, ¾ cup 100
oat bran flakes *(Kellogg's Complete)*, ¾ cup 110
oat bran flakes *(New Morning)*, 1 cup 110
rice *(Kellogg's Rice Krispies)*, 1¼ cup 120
rice *(Kellogg's Smart Start)*, 1 cup 180
rice *(Rice Chex)*, 1¼ cup 120
rice, brown *(New Morning Crispy)*, 1 cup 110
rice, brown, frosted *(New Morning Crispy)*, 1 cup 210
rice, flakes *(Kellogg's Special K)*, 1 cup 110
rice, puffed *(Arrowhead Mills)*, 1 cup 60
spelt flakes *(Arrowhead Mills)*, 1 cup 100
wheat:
    (Kellogg's Frosted Mini-Wheats), 5 pieces 180
    (Kellogg's Frosted Mini-Wheats Bite-Size), 24 pieces . 200
    (Kellogg's Nutri-Grain), ¾ cup 100
    (Nabisco Frosted Wheat Bites), 1 cup 190
    (Wheat Chex), 1 cup 180
    blueberry *(Kellogg's Mini-Wheats)*, ¾ cup 180

Cereal, ready-to-eat, wheat *(cont.)*

flakes *(Wheaties)*, 1 cup 110
puffed *(Arrowhead Mills)*, 1 cup 60
puffed *(Kellogg's Smacks)*, ¾ cup 100
w/raisins *(Crispy Wheaties* 'n Raisins), 1 cup 190
w/raisins *(Kellogg's Raisin Squares)*, ¾ cup 180
raspberry *(Nabisco Fruit Wheats)*, ¾ cup 160
shredded *(Arrowhead Mills)*, 1 cup 180
shredded *(Nabisco)*, 2 biscuits 160
shredded *(Nabisco Spoon Size)*, 1 cup 170
shredded, w/bran *(Nabisco)*, 1¼ cups 200
sweetened *(Honey Frosted Wheaties)*, ¾ cup 110
wheat bran flakes *(Kellogg's Complete)*, ¾ cup 90
wheat bran flakes *(New Morning)*, 1 cup 110
Cereal, cooking/hot (see also specific grains),
uncooked:
barley *(Arrowhead Mills Bits O Barley)*, ⅓ cup 140
barley, banana-nut *(Fantastic Foods* Cup), 1 pkg. 170
farina, see "wheat"
multigrain:
(Arrowhead Mills Instant), 1 pkg. 100
3 grain, maple raisin *(Fantastic Foods* Cup), 1 pkg. . . 180
4 grain w/flax *(Arrowhead Mills)*, ¼ cup 150
7 grain, wheat free *(Arrowhead Mills)*, ¼ cup 120
apple *(Health Valley* Amazing Apple!), 1 pkg. 220
banana nut *(Arrowhead Mills* Instant), 1 pkg. 150
hearty *(Fantastic Foods* Cup), 1 pkg. 260
hearty, w/apricot *(Fantastic Foods* Cup), 1 pkg. 240
maple *(Health Valley* Maple Madness!), 1 pkg. 240
oats/oatmeal:
(H-O Instant/Quick), ½ cup 150
(H-O Regular), 1 pkg. 110
(H-O Oats'n Fiber), 1 pkg. 100
(H-O Power Oats), 1 pkg. 160
apple cinnamon *(Fantastic Foods* Cup), 1 pkg. 170
apple cinnamon *(H-O)*, 1 pkg. 130
cinnamon, raisin, almond *(Arrowhead Mills* Instant),
1 pkg. 130
cranberry orange *(Fantastic Foods* Cup), 1 pkg. 180
maple, apple, spice *(Arrowhead Mills* Instant), 1 pkg. . . 130

maple and brown sugar or raisin-spice *(H-O)*, 1 pkg. . . 160
sweet and mellow *(H-O)*, 1 pkg. 150
rice *(Arrowhead Mills* Instant), 1 pkg. 100
wheat *(Arrowhead Mills Bear Mush)*, ¼ cup 160
wheat, cracked *(Arrowhead Mills)*, ¼ cup 140
wheat, farina *(H-O* Cream), 3 tbsp. 120
wheat and berries *(Fantastic Foods* Cup), 1 pkg. 170
wheat and oats, peachberry *(Fantastic Foods* Cup),
   1 pkg. 190
Cereal crumbs *(Kellogg's* Corn Flakes), 2 tbsp. 40
Cereal bar, see "Granola and cereal bar"
Cereal beverage, see "Coffee substitute"
Chayote, raw *(Frieda's)*, ⅔ cup, 3 oz. 20
Cheese (see also "Cheese Food" and "Cheese
   Spread"), 1 oz., except as noted:
American, processed *(Heluva* Good) 70
American, processed *(Kraft* Deluxe/*Old English* Slices) . . . 110
American, processed *(Kraft* Deluxe/*Old English* Loaf) . . . 100
American, processed *(Land O Lakes* Loaf) 110
American and Swiss *(Land O Lakes* Loaf) 100
blue *(Kraft* Cold Pack/Crumbles) 100
brick *(Land O Lakes)* 100
Brie 95
Camembert 85
cheddar:
   (Boar's Head) 110
   (Kraft) 110
   (Land O Lakes) 110
   mild or sharp *(Kraft Cracker Barrel* ⅓ Less Fat) 80
   mild, sharp, or extra sharp *(Heluva* Good) 110
   nacho blend w/peppers *(Kraft)* 110
   shredded *(Kraft)*, ¼ cup or 1 oz. 120
   shredded, fine *(Kraft)*, ¼ cup or 1 oz. 90
   shredded, mild *(Heluva* Good Reduced Fat) 80
   shredded, mild or sharp *(Heluva* Good) 110
Cheshire 110
chèvre, see "goat," below
Colby *(Boar's Head* Longhorn) 110
Colby *(Kraft)* 110
Colby *(Kraft* ⅓ Less Fat) 80

Cheese *(cont.)*

Colby *(Sargento* Slices) 110
Colby jack *(Kraft)* 110
Colby jack *(Land O Lakes)* 110
Colby jack, shredded *(Kraft),* ¼ cup or 1 oz. 120
cottage, ½ cup:
    4% fat *(Breakstone)* 120
    4% *(Friendship)* 110
    4% *(Friendship* California Style) 115
    4%, w/chives *(Hood)* 110
    4%, w/pineapple *(Friendship)* 140
    4%, w/pineapple *(Hood)* 130
    2% *(Breakstone's)* 90
    2% *(Friendship* Pot Style) 90
    1% *(Hood* Low Fat/No Salt) 80
    1% *(Light n' Lively)* 80
    1%, w/garden salad *(Light n' Lively)* 90
    1%, w/peach and pineapple *(Light n' Lively)* 120
    1%, w/pineapple and cherries *(Hood)* 110
    nonfat *(Friendship)* 80
    nonfat *(Light n' Lively Free)* 80
    nonfat, w/peach or pineapple *(Friendship)* 110
cottage, dry curd *(Breakstone's),* ¼ cup 45
cream cheese *(Boar's Head)* 100
cream cheese *(Philadelphia Brand)* 100
cream cheese *(Philadelphia Brand Free)* 25
cream cheese, w/chives or pimiento *(Philadelphia*
    Brand) 90
cream cheese, soft, 2 tbsp.:
    (Friendship) 100
    (Philadelphia Brand) 100
    (Philadelphia Brand Free) 30
    (Philadelphia Brand Light) 70
    w/chives-onion or herb-garlic *(Philadelphia Brand)* . . . 110
    w/olive-pimiento, pineapple, or salmon *(Philadelphia*
        Brand) 100
cream cheese, whipped *(Breakstone's Temp-Tee),*
    3 tbsp. 110
farmer *(Friendship/Friendship* No Salt) 50
feta *(Athenos)* 80

feta *(Alpine Lace* Reduced Fat) 60
feta, tomato-basil *(Alpine Lace* Reduced Fat) 50
fontina *(Denmark's Finest)* 90
(Gjetost) 130
Glouster, double *(Boar's Head)* 110
goat *(Alpine Lace* Reduced Fat) 40
goat *(Laura Chenel Select* Chèvre) 80
goat, semisoft type 103
Gorgonzola *(Galbani* Dolcelatte) 93
Gouda *(Kraft)* 110
Gruyère 117
havarti *(Kraft)* 120
havarti, all varieties *(Boar's Head)* 110
hoop *(Friendship)* 20
jack, wild morel and leek *(Great Midwest)* 100
jalapeño jack *(Land O Lakes)* 100
(Jarlsberg) 100
Limburger *(Kraft)* 90
Monterey jack, plain or w/jalapeño *(Kraft)* 110
Monterey jack, plain or w/peppers *(Kraft* ⅓ Less Fat) 80
Monterey jack, plain or w/jalapeño *(Boar's Head)* 100
Monterey jack, shredded *(Kraft),* ¼ cup or 1 oz. 110
mozzarella *(Sargento* Slices) 130
mozzarella *(Sargento Preferred Light* Slices) 90
mozzarella, whole milk *(Heluva* Good) 100
mozzarella, part skim *(Kraft)* 80
mozzarella, part skim *(Land O Lakes)* 80
mozzarella, shredded *(Kraft),* ¼ cup or 1 oz. 90
Muenster *(Boar's Head)* 100
Muenster *(Kraft)* 110
Meunster *(Land O Lakes)* 100
Neufchâtel *(Philadelphia Brand)* 70
Parmesan, grated *(Di Giorno),* 2 tsp. 20
Parmesan, grated *(Kraft* 100%), 2 tsp. 20
Parmesan, grated *(Sargento),* 1 tbsp. 25
Parmesan, shredded *(Kraft* 100%), 2 tsp. 20
Parmesan and Romano, grated *(Sargento),* 1 tbsp. 25
pizza blend, shredded *(Sargento),* ¼ cup or 1 oz. 90
Port du Salut 100
provolone *(Boar's Head* Picante/Sharp) 100

Cheese *(cont.)*

provolone *(Land O Lakes)* 100
ricotta *(Breakstone's)*, ¼ cup 110
ricotta *(Sargento* Light), ¼ cup 60
ricotta *(Sargento* Old Fashioned), ¼ cup 90
ricotta, part skim *(Sargento)*, ¼ cup 80
Romano, grated *(Di Giorno* 100%), 2 tsp. 25
Romano, grated or shredded *(Di Giorno)*, 2 tsp. 20
Roquefort 105
Swiss *(Boar's Head* Baby/Gold Label Imported) 110
Swiss *(Kraft/Kraft* Baby) 110
Swiss, light *(Land O Lakes* 50% Reduced Fat) 80
Swiss, processed *(Kraft* Deluxe), 1-oz. slice 90
Swiss, shredded *(Kraft)*, ¼ cup or 1 oz. 110

"Cheese," substitute and nondairy:

(Smart Beat Lactose Free), ⅔-oz. slice 25
American *(Smart Beat)*, ⅔-oz slice 25
American, shredded *(Harvest Moon)*, ¼ cup 120
cheddar, mellow or sharp *(Smart Beat)*, ⅔-oz. slice . . . 25
cheddar, shredded *(Harvest Moon)*, ¼ cup 120
mozzarella, shredded *(Harvest Moon)*, ¼ cup or 1 oz. . . 110

Cheese dip, 2 tbsp., except as noted:

blue *(Kraft* Premium) 45
blue *(T. Marzetti's* Dip & Dressing) 150
cheddar *(Frito-Lay* Mild) 60
cheddar, w/jalapeño *(Breakstone's)* 60
cheddar, w/jalapeño *(Frito-Lay)* 50
w/chili *(Fritos)* 45
jalapeño *(Kraft* Premium) 60
nacho *(Frito-Lay)* 45
nacho *(Kraft* Premium) 60
nacho, w/beef *(Tostitos)*, 4 tbsp. 120
salsa *(Heluva* Good Cheese 'N Salsa) 80
salsa *(Old El Paso)* 40
salsa *(Old El Paso* Chunky/Low Fat) 30
salsa *(Tostitos)*, 4 tbsp. 80

Cheese food (see also "Cheese" and "Cheese
    spreads"):

all varieties *(Kraft* Singles), ¾-oz. slice 70
American, grated *(Kraft)*, 1 tbsp. 25

cheddar *(Cracker Barrel)*, 2 tbsp. 100
w/garlic *(Kraft)*, 1 oz. 90
herb, onion, pepperoni, or salami *(Land O Lakes)*, 1 oz. . . 90
w/jalapeño *(Kraft)*, 1 oz. 90
shredded *(Velveeta)*, ¼ cup 130
Swiss *(Kraft* Singles), ¾-oz. slice 70
Cheese pocket, grilled, frozen *(Hot Pockets Toaster*
   Breaks), 2.1-oz. piece 210
Cheese and pretzels, see "Pretzels"
Cheese product (see also "Cheese food"):
(Kraft Free Singles), ⅔-oz. slice 30
(Velveeta Light), 1 oz. 60
American flavor *(Kraft* Deluxe 25% Less Fat), ¾-oz.
   slice 70
cheddar flavor, sharp *(Kraft* Singles ⅓ Less Fat), ¾-oz.
   slice 50
cheddar flavor sharp *(Kraft Free* Singles), ¾-oz. slice . . . 30
mozzarella flavor *(Alpine Lace* Fat Free Loaf) 45
Swiss *(Kraft* Singles ⅓ Less Fat), ¾-oz. slice 50
Swiss *(Kraft Free* Singles), ¾-oz. slice 30
Cheese puffs, see "Cake, snack"
Cheese sauce, 2 tbsp.:
(Cheez Whiz Zap-A-Pack) 90
picante *(Pace* Con Queso) 90
Cheese sauce, cooking, in jars, ¼ cup:
Alfredo *(Ragú Cheese Creations!* Classic) 120
Alfredo, light Parmesan *(Ragú Cheese Creations!)* 80
cheddar, double *(Ragú Cheese Creations!)* 110
cheddar and tomato, spicy *(Ragú Cheese Creations!)* 50
four cheese or roasted garlic *(Ragú Cheese Creations!)* . . 120
Romano, cream tomato *(Ragú Cheese Creations!)* 60
Cheese spread (see also "Cheese"), 2 tbsp., except as
   noted:
(Cheez Whiz Light) 80
(Cheez Whiz Squeezable) 100
(Land O Lakes Golden Velvet), 1 oz. 80
(Squeez-A-Snak) 90
(Velveeta/Velveeta Italiana), 1 oz. 80
all varieties *(Cheez Whiz)* 90
American *(Easy Cheese)* 100

Cheese spread *(cont.)*
American *(Harvest Moon)*, ⅔ oz. 50
w/bacon *(Kraft)* 90
blue cheese *(Kraft Roka)* 80
cheddar *(Easy Cheese)* 100
cheddar, medium or sharp *(Spreadery)* 80
cheddar, plain or bacon/horseradish *(Heluva* Good Cold
  Pack) 90
garlic herb *(Alpine Lace* Reduced Fat) 60
w/jalapeño *(Kraft* Loaf), 1 oz. 80
w/jalapeño, hot or mild *(Velveeta)*, 1 oz. 80
Limburger *(Mohawk Valley)* 80
Neufchâtel, garden vegetable *(Spreadery)* 70
Neufchâtel, garlic, herb, or ranch *(Spreadery)* 80
olive and pimiento or pineapple *(Kraft)* 70
pimiento *(Kraft)* 80
pimiento *(Spreadery)* 100
port wine *(Heluva* Good Cold Pack) 90
slices *(Velveeta)*, ¾-oz. slice 60
sundried tomato-basil *(Alpine Lace* Reduced Fat) 70
Cheese sticks, frozen, breaded, w/sauce, 2 pieces,
  except as noted:
jalapeño cheddar *(Rich-SeaPak* Fiesta Dippers) 140
jalapeño cream cheese *(Rich-SeaPak* Fiesta Dippers) . . . 130
Italian 4-cheese *(Rich-SeaPak* Dippers) 140
mozzarella *(Rich-SeaPak* Dippers) 190
mozzarella, w/out sauce *(Banquet)*, 6 pieces 280
pizza, double cheese *(Rich-SeaPak* Dippers), approx. 3
  pieces 210
pizza, pepperoni *(Rich-SeaPak* Dippers), approx.
  3 pieces 230
Cherimoya *(Frieda's)*, 5 oz. 130
Cherry, ½ cup, except as noted:
fresh, sour, red, w/pits 26
fresh, sweet, w/pits 52
fresh, sweet, 10 medium, 2.6 oz. 49
canned, sour, pitted, in heavy syrup 116
canned, sweet, pitted, dark, in heavy syrup *(Del Monte)* . 100
Cherry, dried, bing *(Frieda's)*, ¼ cup, 1.4 oz. 120
Cherry, maraschino, w/liquid, 1 oz. 33

Cherry, maraschino, syrup *(Trader Vic's)*, 1 fl. oz. 90
Cherry drink *(Ocean Spray Black Cherry Blast)*, 8 fl. oz. . . 140
Cherry juice *(Dole* Mountain), 8 fl. oz. 150
Chervil, dried, 1 tsp. 1
Chestnut, Chinese, shelled, boiled, or steamed, 1 oz. 44
Chestnut, European:
boiled, 1 oz. 37
roasted, peeled, 1 oz. 70
roasted, peeled, 1 cup, 17 kernels 350
roasted, peeled, in jars *(Minerve),* 4 whole, 1.1 oz. 50
Chestnut, Japanese, dried, 1 oz. 102
Chicken, fresh, 4 oz., except as noted:
broiler-fryer, roasted:
   w/skin, ½ chicken, 10½ oz. (15.8 oz. w/bone) 715
   w/skin 271
   meat only 215
   meat only, chopped or diced, 1 cup 266
   skin only, 1 oz. 129
   dark meat only 232
   light meat only 196
   breast, w/skin, ½ breast, 3½ oz. (8½ oz. w/bone) . . . 193
   drumstick, w/skin, 1.8 oz. (2.9 oz. w/bone) 112
   leg, w/skin (5.7 oz. w/bone) 265
   thigh, w/skin, 2.2 oz. (2.9 oz. w/bone) 153
   wing, w/skin, 1.2 oz. (2.3 oz. w/bone) 99
capon, roasted, w/skin, ½ capon, 1.4 lbs. (2 lbs. w/
  bone) 1457
capon, roasted, w/skin 260
Cornish hen, see "Cornish hen"
roaster, roasted, w/skin, ½ chicken, 1 lb. (1½ lbs. w/
  bone) 1071
roaster, roasted, meat w/skin 253
stewing, stewed, meat only 269
Chicken, canned, chunk, in water *(Swanson* Premium),
  2 oz. 60
Chicken, frozen or refrigerated, cooked (see also
  "Chicken entree, frozen"):
breast, crispy baked, 1 piece, 3.5 oz.:
   (Butterball Chicken Requests Original) 180

Chicken, frozen or refrigerated, cooked, breast *(cont.)*

Italian herb or lemon peppper *(Butterball Chicken
Requests)* 190

Parmesan *(Butterball Chicken Requests)* 200

Southwestern *(Butterball Chicken Requests)* 170

breast, oven-roasted *(Tyson)* 2 oz. 80

breast fillet, breaded *(Tyson)*, 2 pieces, 2.9 oz. 180

breast fillet, Southern fried *(Tyson)*, 2 pieces, 3.5 oz. . . . 210

breast strips *(Tyson)*, 3 oz. 90

breast strips, seasoned *(Tyson)*, 3 oz. 140

breast strips, Southwestern *(Tyson)*, 3 oz. 110

breast tenders:

(Banquet Original), 3 pieces 240

baked *(Banquet* Fat Free), 3 pieces 120

baked *(Butterball Chicken Requests)*, 3 pieces 170

w/barbecue sauce *(Banquet)*, 3 pieces 340

breaded *(Tyson)*, 5 pieces, 3 oz. 220

breaded *(Tyson* Tenderloins), 2 pieces, 3.2 oz. 180

breaded, honey batter *(Tyson)*, 5 pieces, 3 oz. 200

breaded, patties *(Tyson)*, 3 pieces, 3.2 oz. 100

Southern *(Banquet)*, 3 pieces 260

chunks, breaded *(Tyson)*, 6 pieces, 3 oz. 220

chunks, breaded, Southern *(Banquet)*, 5 pieces 270

chunks, breaded, Southern *(Tyson)*, 6 pieces, 3 oz. 260

drumsticks, barbecue, hot *(Tyson)*, 2 pieces, 3.5 oz. 160

fried, bone-in, 3 oz., except as noted:

(Banquet Original) 280

(Banquet Original Jumbo Pack) 270

breasts *(Banquet* Original), 5.5-oz. piece 410

country *(Banquet)* 270

drums and thighs *(Banquet)* 260

honey barbecue, skinless *(Banquet)* 230

hot and spicy *(Banquet)* 260

lemon pepper, skinless *(Banquet)* 210

Southern *(Banquet)* 280

wings, hot and spicy *(Banquet)*, 4 pieces 260

grilled, lemon pepper fillet *(Tyson)*, 1 piece, 2.7 oz. 100

nuggets *(Banquet* Original), 6 pieces 270

nuggets *(Tyson)*, 4 pieces, 3.8 oz. 240

nuggets *(Tyson)*, 3-oz. piece 220

nuggets, w/sauce, see "Chicken entree, frozen"
patty, breaded, 1 piece:
    (Banquet Fat Free) 100
    (Banquet Original) 190
    (Tyson) 190
    (Tyson Thick'n Crispy) 200
    breast *(Tyson)* 80
    cheddar *(Tyson* Chick'n Quick Chick'n Cheddar) 220
    Southern *(Banquet)* 170
    nugget shape *(Tyson),* 6 pieces, 3.8 oz. 250
    Southern, breast *(Tyson)* 180
patties, mesquite *(Tyson),* 1 piece, 2.8 oz. 110
shredded, w/barbecue sauce *(Lloyd's),* ¼ cup 70
wing *(Tyson* Wings of Fire), 3 pieces, 3.4 oz. 220
wing, barbecue *(Tyson),* 3 pieces, 3.2 oz. 200
wing, *Tabasco (Tyson),* 3 pieces, 2.7 oz. 170
wing, teriyaki *(Tyson),* 4 pieces, 3.4 oz. 190
Chicken, ground, raw *(Perdue),* 4 oz. 180
"Chicken," vegetarian, frozen:
(Worthington Chic-Ketts), 2 slices, ⅜″ 120
(Worthington ChikStiks), 1 piece 110
nuggets *(Loma Linda),* 5 pieces 240
nuggets *(Morningstar Farms),* 4 pieces 160
patty *(Morningstar Farms* Chik), 1 patty 150
patty *(Worthington CrispyChik),* 1 patty 150
slice or roll *(Morningstar Farms),* 2 slices 80
Chicken dinner, frozen, 1 pkg.:
breaded, country *(Healthy Choice),* 10.25 oz. 350
broccoli Alfredo *(Healthy Choice),* 11.5 oz. 300
cacciatore *(Healthy Choice),* 12.5 oz. 270
Cantonese *(Healthy Choice),* 10.75 oz. 280
Dijon *(Healthy Choice),* 11 oz. 270
Francesca *(Healthy Choice),* 12.5 oz. 330
fried *(Banquet Extra Helping),* 18 oz. 910
fried, country, w/gravy *(Marie Callender's),* 16 oz. 620
ginger Hunan *(Healthy Choice),* 12.6 oz. 350
grilled, mushroom sauce *(Marie Callender's),* 14 oz. . . . 480
grilled, Southwestern *(Healthy Choice),* 10.2 oz. 260
herb, country *(Healthy Choice),* 12.15 oz. 320
mesquite, barbecue *(Healthy Choice),* 10.5 oz. 310

Chicken dinner, frozen *(cont.)*

parmigiana *(Healthy Choice)*, 11.5 oz. 330
parmigiana *(Marie Callender's)*, 16 oz. 620
picante *(Healthy Choice)*, 10.75 oz. 260
roasted *(Healthy Choice)*, 11 oz. 230
sesame, Shanghai *(Healthy Choice)*, 12 oz. 300
sweet and sour *(Healthy Choice)*, 11 oz. 360
sweet and sour *(Marie Callender's)*, 14 oz. 530
teriyaki *(Healthy Choice)*, 11 oz. 270

Chicken entree, frozen (see also "Chicken, frozen or refrigerated, cooked"), 1 pkg., except as noted:

à la king *(Stouffer's)*, 9½ oz. 350
Alfredo *(Stouffer's Skillet Sensations)*, ½ of 25-oz. pkg. . 490
baked *(Lean Cuisine American Favorites)*, 8⅝ oz. 230
barbecue, w/potato, vegetables *(Tyson)*, 14.8 oz. 560
barbecue, *Tabasco* sauce *(Tyson)*, 9 oz. 260
barbecue sauce *(Lean Cuisine Hearty Portions)*, 13⅞ oz. . 380
w/basil cream sauce *(Lean Cuisine Cafe Classics)*,
   8½ oz. 270
blackened, w/rice, corn *(Tyson)*, 9 oz. 260
breast, baked *(Stouffer's Homestyle)*, 8⅞ oz. 260
breast, in barbecue sauce *(Stouffer's Homestyle)*, 10 oz. . 510
breast, w/mushroom gravy *(Stouffer's Homestyle)*,
   10 oz. 360
breast, in wine sauce *(Lean Cuisine Cafe Classics)*,
   8⅛ oz. 210
and broccoli *(Healthy Choice Hearty Handfuls)*, 6.1 oz. . . . 320
and broccoli, w/cheese, carrots, pasta *(Tyson)*, 9 oz. . . . 270
carbonara *(Lean Cuisine Cafe Classics)*, 9 oz. 280
chow mein, w/egg rolls *(Banquet Meal)*, 9 oz. 210
chow mein, w/rice *(Lean Cuisine)*, 9 oz. 220
chow mein, w/rice *(Stouffer's)*, 10⅝ oz. 220
Cordon Bleu *(Marie Callender's)*, 13 oz. 590
creamed *(Stouffer's)*, 6½ oz. 260
divan, w/carrots, pasta *(Tyson)*, 10 oz. 370
and dumplings *(Stouffer's Homestyle)*, 11 oz. 280
and dumplings, w/gravy *(Banquet Meal)*, 10 oz. 270
enchilada, see "Enchilada"
fajita *(Healthy Choice Fiesta)*, 7 oz. 260
fajita *(Tyson)*, 3½ pieces, 13.2 oz. 460

fettuccine *(Lean Cuisine)*, 9¼ oz. 300
fettuccine *(Stouffer's* Homestyle), 10½ oz. 350
fettuccine *(Stouffer's Hearty Portions)*, 16¾ oz. 640
fettuccine Alfredo *(Banquet* Meal), 10.25 oz. 420
fettuccine Alfredo *(Healthy Choice)*, 8.5 oz. 260
Florentine *(Lean Cuisine Hearty Portions)*, 13¼ oz. 440
fiesta *(Lean Cuisine Cafe Classics)*, 8½ oz. 270
fingers, w/barbecue sauce *(Banquet* Meal), 9 oz. 340
Français, w/red potato, green beans *(Tyson)*, 9 oz. 260
fried *(Banquet* Meal Original), 9 oz. 470
fried, breast *(Stouffer's* Homestyle), 8⅞ oz. 400
fried, breast *(Stouffer's Hearty Portions)*, 15 oz. 500
fried, w/gravy, w/mashed potato *(Tyson)*, 10.9 oz. 360
fried, Southern *(Banquet* Meal), 8.75 oz. 560
fried, white meat *(Banquet* Meal), 8.75 oz. 480
garlic *(Healthy Choice Hearty Handfuls)*, 6.1 oz. 330
garlic Milano *(Healthy Choice)*, 9.5 oz. 240
glazed *(Lean Cuisine Cafe Classics)*, 8½ oz. 240
glazed, country *(Healthy Choice)*, 8½ oz. 230
glazed, w/rice *(Stouffer's)*, ⅕ of 59-oz. pkg. 290
grilled *(Lean Cuisine Cafe Classics)*, 8⅞ oz. 260
grilled, w/corn O'Brien, beans *(Tyson)*, 9 oz. 230
grilled, Italian, w/pasta, vegetables *(Tyson)*, 9 oz. 190
grilled, w/mashed potatoes *(Healthy Choice)*, 8 oz. 170
grilled, and penne *(Lean Cuisine Hearty Portions)*,
    14 oz. 380
grilled, salsa *(Lean Cuisine Cafe Classics)*, 8⅞ oz. 270
grilled, Sonoma *(Healthy Choice)*, 9 oz. 230
herb roasted *(Lean Cuisine Cafe Classics)*, 8 oz. 200
herb roasted, w/mashed potato *(Marie Callender's)*,
    14 oz. 670
homestyle *(Stouffer's Skillet Sensations)*, ½ of 25-oz.
    pkg. 390
honey mustard *(Healthy Choice)*, 9.5 oz. 270
honey mustard *(Lean Cuisine Cafe Classics)*, 8 oz. 260
imperial *(Healthy Choice)*, 9 oz. 230
honey Dijon, w/pasta, peas *(Tyson)*, 11.4 oz. 340
honey roasted *(Lean Cuisine American Favorites)*,
    8½ oz. 270
Kiev, w/rice pilaf, broccoli, and carrots *(Tyson)*, 9 oz. . . . 440

Chicken entree, frozen *(cont.)*
mandarin *(Healthy Choice)*, 10 oz. 280
mandarin *(Lean Cuisine)*, 9 oz. 250
Marsala *(Marie Callender's)*, 14 oz. 450
Marsala, w/vegetables *(Healthy Choice)*, 11.5 oz. 240
medallions *(Lean Cuisine American Favorites)*, 9⅜ oz. . . . 260
Mediterranean *(Lean Cuisine Cafe Classics)*, 10½ oz. . . . 260
mesquite, w/corn, peas, au gratin potato *(Tyson)*, 9 oz. . 320
and mushroom *(Healthy Choice Hearty Handfuls)*,
    6.1 oz. 310
w/mushroom sauce, rice pilaf, carrots *(Tyson)*, 9 oz. 220
and noodles *(Marie Callender's)*, 13 oz. 520
and noodles, escalloped *(Stouffer's)*, 10 oz. 460
nuggets, Southern, w/barbecue sauce *(Banquet* Micro),
    6 pieces 340
nuggets, w/sweet and sour sauce *(Banquet* Micro),
    6 pieces 320
à l'orange *(Lean Cuisine Cafe Classics)*, 9 oz. 260
Oriental *(Lean Cuisine Skillet Sensations)*, ½ of 24-oz.
    pkg. 280
Oriental, w/egg rolls *(Banquet)*, 9 oz. 260
Oriental, glazed *(Lean Cuisine Hearty Portions)*, 14 oz. . . . 350
Parmesan *(Lean Cuisine Cafe Classics)*, 10⅞ oz. 260
parmigiana *(Banquet* Meal), 9.5 oz. 320
parmigiana *(Stouffer's* Homestyle), 12 oz. 460
pasta fiesta *(Marie Callender's)*, 12.5 oz. 640
pasta primavera *(Banquet* Meal), 9.5 oz. 320
in peanut sauce *(Lean Cuisine Cafe Classics)*, 9 oz. 290
penne, rosemary *(Tyson* Kit), 12.5 oz. 330
piccata *(Lean Cuisine Cafe Classics)*, 9 oz. 270
piccata *(Tyson)*, 9 oz. 190
pie *(Banquet)*, 7-oz. pie 380
pie *(Lean Cuisine)*, 9½-oz. pie 290
pie *(Marie Callender's)*, 9.5-oz. pie 600
pie *(Stouffer's)*, 10-oz. pie 490
pie *(Stouffer's Hearty Portions)*, 16 oz. 590
pie, au gratin *(Marie Callender's)*, 9.5-oz. pie 690
pie, and broccoli *(Banquet)*, 7-oz. pie 330
pie, and broccoli *(Marie Callender's)*, 9.5-oz. pie 670

primavera *(Lean Cuisine Skillet Sensations)*, ½ of 24-oz.
   pkg. 320
primavera *(Tyson)*, 11.4 oz. 350
rice, cheesy, w/chicken and broccoli *(Marie Callender's)*,
   12 oz. 390
rice, fried *(Tyson* Kit), 14 oz., 2½ cups 440
roasted, w/garlic sauce, pasta, vegetables *(Tyson)*, 9 oz. . 210
roasted, w/mushrooms *(Lean Cuisine Hearty Portions)*,
   12½ oz. 340
tenderloins, in gravy w/potatoes *(Stouffer's)*, ⅕ of
   61-oz. pkg. 330
teriyaki *(Stouffer's Skillet Sensations)*, ½ of 25-oz. pkg. . 340
sesame *(Healthy Choice)*, 9.75 oz. 240
stir-fry *(Tyson* Kit), 14 oz., 2¾ cups 430
and vegetables *(Lean Cuisine Cafe Classics)*, 10½ oz. . . . 270
and vegetables *(Stouffer's Skillet Sensations)*, ½ of
   25-oz. pkg. 440
Chicken entree mix, stir-fry *(Skillet Chicken Helper)*,
   1 cup* 270
Chicken fat, rendered *(Empire* Kosher), 1 tbsp. 120
Chicken giblets, simmered, chopped, 1 cup 228
Chicken gravy, canned, ¼ cup:
(Franco-American) 40
(Franco-American Fat Free) 15
(Franco-American Slow Roasted) 25
(Franco-American Slow Roasted Fat Free) 20
giblet *(Franco-American)* 30
Chicken gravy mix, style *(Pillsbury)*, ¼ cup* 20
Chicken lunch meat, breast:
barbecue *(Black Bear)*, 2 oz. 70
browned *(Healthy Choice)*, 2 oz. 60
honey *(Tyson* Fat Free), 2 slices, 1.5 oz. 35
mesquite *(Healthy Choice)*, 2 oz. 60
mesquite *(Tyson* Fat Free), 2 slices, 1.5 oz. 35
oven-roasted *(Boar's Head)*, 2 oz. 50
oven-roasted *(Healthy Choice)*, 1-oz. slice 25
oven-roasted *(Healthy Choice* 10 oz.), 1-oz. slice 35
oven-roasted *(Healthy Choice* Deli-Thin), 6 slices,
   1.8 oz. 60

Chicken lunch meat *(cont.)*
oven-roasted or peppered *(Tyson* Fat Free), 2 slices,
  1.5 oz. 35
rotisserie *(Healthy Choice* Hearty Deli), 3 slices, 2 oz. 60
smoked *(Healthy Choice),* 1-oz. slice 30
smoked, hickory *(Boar's Head),* 2 oz. 60
smoked, hickory *(Tyson* Fat Free), 2 slices, 1.5 oz. 35
white meat *(Tyson),* 2 slices, 1.3 oz. 60
white meat, rolled *(Tyson),* 2 oz. 90
Chicken patty, see "Chicken, frozen, cooked"
Chicken pie, see "Chicken entree, frozen"
Chicken pocket, frozen, 4.5-oz. piece:
broccoli *(Lean Pockets* Supreme) 270
broccoli and cheddar *(Croissant Pockets)* 290
and cheddar w/broccoli *(Hot Pockets)* 300
Parmesan *(Lean Pockets).* 280
Chicken sandwich, frozen, 1 piece:
breast *(Tyson* Microwave), 4.2 oz. 320
grilled *(Tyson* Microwave), 3.5 oz. 210
Chicken sauce (see also specific listings):
cacciatore *(Chicken Tonight),* ½ cup 70
Dijon, country *(Lawry's Chicken Saute),* 2 tbsp. 40
French, country *(Chicken Tonight),* ½ cup 120
honey mustard, light *(Chicken Tonight),* ½ cup 60
lemon herb *(Lawry's Chicken Saute),* 2 tbsp. 25
mushroom, creamy *(Chicken Tonight),* ½ cup 80
sweet and sour *(Chicken Tonight),* ½ cup 120
Chicken sausage, see "Sausage"
Chicken seasoning and coating mix, ⅛ pkg.:
(Shake'n Bake Original/Hot and Spicy) 40
barbecue *(Shake'n Bake)* 45
extra crispy *(Oven Fry)* 60
homestyle flour *(Oven Fry)* 40
Chicken spread *(Underwood),* ¼ cup 120
Chick-fil-A, 1 serving:
chicken soup, hearty breast of, 1 cup 110
chicken dishes:
    chargrilled chicken garden salad 170
    chicken salad plate 290
    Chick-fil-A Nuggets, 8-pack 290

Chick-fil-A Chick-n-Strips, 4 pieces 230
   Chick-n-Strips salad 290
Chick-fil-A sandwich:
   regular. 290
   deluxe 300
   chicken only, no bun/pickles 160
Chick-fil-A Chargrilled Chicken Sandwich:
   regular. 280
   deluxe 290
   club, w/out dressing 390
   chicken only, no bun/pickles 130
Chick-fil-A chicken salad sandwich, on whole wheat 320
side items, small:
   carrot-raisin salad 150
   cole slaw 130
   Chick-fil-A Waffle Potato Fries 290
   tossed salad 70
desserts:
   brownie, fudge nut 350
   cheesecake, slice 270
   cheesecake, w/blueberry or strawberry 290
   Icedream, small cone 140
   Icedream, small cup 350
   lemon pie, slice 320
Chickpeas, see "Garbanzo beans"
Chicory, witloof:
(*Frieda's* Belgium Endive), 2 cups, 3 oz. 15
5–7″ head, 2.1 oz. 9
Chicory greens, chopped, ½ cup 21
Chili, canned, 1 cup, except as noted:
w/beans (*El Rio*) 240
w/beans (*Old El Paso*) 240
w/black beans (*El Rio*) 220
w/black beans, mild (*Arrowhead Mills*) 190
w/black beans, spicy (*Arrowhead Mills*) 200
vegetarian (*Arrowhead Mills* Panhandle) 200
vegetarian, all varieties (*Health Valley*), ½ cup 80
vegetarian, mild, medium or hot (*Muir Glen*) 150
Chili, frozen, see "Chili dinner" and "Chili entree"

Chili, mix, all varieties *(Health Valley* Chili in a Cup),
¾ cup 120
Chili beans (see also "Mexican beans"), canned, ½
cup:
all varieties *(Brooks)*. 130
spicy *(Green Giant/Joan of Arc)* 110
zesty sauce *(Campbell's)* 130
Chili dinner, frozen, black bean *(Amy's),* 10.5 oz. 320
Chili dip (see also "Salsa"), chunky *(La Victoria),*
2 tbsp. 10
Chili dishes, mix, 1 pkg.:
black bean, w/corn *(Fantastic Foods Chile Ole!* Cup) 250
mac, w/ziti *(Fantastic Foods Chile Ole!* Cup) 270
nacho, w/tortillas *(Fantastic Foods Chile Ole!* Cup) 260
white bean, spicy *(Fantastic Foods Chile Ole!* Cup) 260
Chili entree, frozen:
w/beans *(Stouffer's),* 8¾ oz. 270
3-bean, w/rice *(Lean Cuisine),* 10 oz. 250
and cornbread *(Marie Callender's),* 1 cup, 2 oz.
cornbread 350
Chili pepper, see "Pepper, chili"
Chili powder, 1 tbsp. 24
Chili sauce, tomato (see also "Pepper sauce"), 1 tbsp.:
(Del Monte). 20
(Heinz) 15
Chili seasoning mix *(Old El Paso),* 1 tbsp. 15
Chimichanga, frozen:
beef *(Old El Paso),* 4.5-oz. piece 360
chicken *(Old El Paso),* 4.5-oz. piece 340
Chitterlings, pork, simmered, 4 oz. 344
Chives, fresh or freeze-dried, chopped, 1 tbsp. 1
Chocolate, see "Candy"
Chocolate, baking:
(Choco Bake), ½ oz. 80
bar *(Baker's German),* ½ oz. 60
bar *(Hershey's),* ½ of 1-oz. bar 90
bar, bittersweet or dark *(Ghirardelli),* 3 pieces, 1.5 oz. . . . 210
bar, bittersweet or semisweet *(Hershey's),* ½ of 1-oz.
bar 70
bar, milk *(Ghirardelli),* 3 pieces, 1.5 oz. 220

bar, semisweet *(Baker's)*, 1 oz. 130
bar, semisweet *(Nestlé)*, ½ oz. 70
bar, unsweetened *(Baker's)*, 1 oz. 140
bar, unsweetened or white *(Nestlé)*, ½ oz. 80
bar, white *(Baker's)*, 1 oz. 160
bits, holiday *(Hershey's)*, 1 tbsp. 70
chips or morsels, 1 tbsp. or ½ oz.:
    all varieties *(Hershey's)* 80
    milk or mint *(Nestlé)* 70
    semisweet *(Baker's)* 60
    semisweet *(Hershey's Lowfat)* 60
    semisweet *(Nestlé/Nestlé Mini/Nestlé Mega)* 70
    white *(Nestlé)* 80
kisses *(Hershey's Mini)*, 11 pieces 80
Chocolate dip, for fruit *(Smucker's Fat Free)*, 2 tbsp. . . . 130
Chocolate drink *(Yoo-Hoo)*, 9 fl. oz. 150
Chocolate drink mix *(Nestlé Quik)*, 4 tbsp. 100
Chocolate milk, dairy, 1 cup:
(Hershey's Lowfat) 190
(Hood 1% Lowfat) 170
Chocolate shake *(Hershey's)*, 7 fl. oz. 230
Chocolate sprinkles *(Hershey's Chocolate Shoppe)*,
    2 tbsp. 140
Chocolate syrup, 2 tbsp.:
dark *(Hershey's Special Dark)* 110
regular or malt *(Hershey's)* 100
Chocolate topping, 2 tbsp.:
(Kraft) 110
all varieties *(Hershey's Fat Free)* 100
dark *(Dove)* 140
fudge *(Smucker's/Smucker's Microwave)* 130
fudge, hot *(Kraft)* 140
fudge, hot *(Smucker's/Smucker's Special Recipe)* 140
fudge, hot *(Smucker's Light)* 90
fudge, hot *(Smucker's Microwave)* 130
fudge, hot *(Smucker's Microwave Fat Free)* 110
milk *(Dove)* 130
nut *(Smucker's Magic Shell)* 220
Chorizo, see "Sausage"

Chutney:
(Crosse & Blackwell Major Grey's/Hot Mango), 1 tbsp. 60
(Trader Vic's Calcutta), 2 tbsp. 44
apple curry *(Crosse & Blackwell)*, 1 tbsp. 25
cranberry *(Crosse & Blackwell)*, 1 tbsp. 40
Cilantro, see "Coriander"
Cinnamon, ground, 1 tsp. 6
Cisco, meat only, raw, 4 oz. 112
Citrus drink blend:
(Tropicana), 8 fl. oz. 140
(Tropicana Twister), 10 fl. oz. 180
(V8 Splash), 8 fl. oz. 120
Clam, meat only:
raw, 4 oz. 84
raw, 9 large or 20 small, 6.3 oz. 133
boiled, poached, or steamed, 4 oz. 168
Clam, canned, ¼ cup or 2 oz.:
chopped, ocean *(Chincoteague)* 30
chopped, sea, Eastern *(Chincoteague)* 25
minced *(Progresso)*, ¼ cup 25
Clam, fried, frozen:
(Mrs. Paul's), 4.5-oz. pkg. 370
(Van de Kamp's), 5-oz. pkg. 410
Clam chowder, see "Soup"
Clam dip, 2 tbsp.:
(Heluva Good New England) 50
(Kraft) 60
(Kraft Premium) 45
Chesapeake *(Breakstone's)* 50
Clam juice, 8 fl. oz.:
ocean *(Chincoteague)* 10
sea *(Chincoteague)* 15
Clam sauce, canned, ½ cup:
red *(Progresso)* 60
white *(Chincoteague)* 120
white *(Progresso)* 140
white *(Progresso* Authentic) 150
white *(Rienzi)* 130
white, creamy *(Progresso)* 110
Cloves, ground, 1 tsp. 7

Cobbler, frozen:

apple *(Mrs. Smith's)*, ⅛ cobbler, 4 oz. 240
apple cinnamon or crumb *(Pet-Ritz)*, ⅙ cobbler, 4.3 oz. . 280
blackberry *(Mrs. Smith's)*, ⅛ cobbler, 4 oz. 250
blackberry *(Pet-Ritz)*, ⅙ cobbler, 4.3 oz. 260
blackberry crumb *(Pet-Ritz)*, ⅙ cobbler, 4.3 oz. 260
cherry *(Mrs. Smith's)*, ⅛ cobbler, 4 oz. 250
cherry *(Pet-Ritz)*, ⅙ cobbler, 4.3 oz. 300
cherry crumb *(Pet-Ritz)*, ⅙ cobbler, 4.3 oz. 280
peach *(Mrs. Smith's)*, ⅛ cobbler, 4 oz. 240
peach *(Pet-Ritz)*, ⅙ cobbler, 4.3 oz. 240
peach crumb *(Pet-Ritz)*, ⅙ cobbler, 4.3 oz. 230
strawberry *(Pet-Ritz)*, ⅙ cobbler, 4.3 oz. 260
Cocktail sauce, see "Seafood sauce"
Cocoa, baking, unsweetened:
(Ghirardelli), 1 tbsp. 35
(Hershey's/Hershey's European Style), 1 tbsp. 20
(Nestlé), 1 tbsp. 15
Cocoa mix, hot, 1 pkt., except as noted:
chocolate, almond or amaretto *(Hershey's)* 150
chocolate, double, hazelnut, or mocha *(Ghirardelli)* 90
chocolate, Dutch *(Hershey's)* 160
chocolate, mint or raspberry *(Hershey's)* 150
Irish creme *(Hershey's)* 150
Swiss mocha or French vanilla *(Hershey's)* 140
Cocoa-coffee mix *(Trader Vic's* Kafe-La-Te), ½ oz. 50
Coconut:
fresh, shelled, 1 oz. 100
dried, toasted, 1 oz. 168
packaged, flaked *(Baker's Angel Flake)*, 2 tbsp. 70
packaged *(Baker's* Premium Shred), 2 tbsp. 60
packaged *(Mounds)*, 2 tbsp. 70
Coconut cream, canned, 1 tbsp. 36
Cod, meat only:
Atlantic, raw, 4 oz. 93
Atlantic, bake, broiled, or microwaved, 4 oz. 119
Pacific, raw, 4 oz. 93
Pacific, baked, broiled, or microwaved, 4 oz. 119
Cod, dried, Atlantic, salted, 1 oz. 81

Cod entree, frozen:

au gratin *(Oven Poppers),* 5-oz. piece 220

fillets, breaded *(Mrs. Paul's),* 1 piece 250

fillets, breaded *(Van de Kamp's),* 1 piece 220

stuffed w/broccoli, cheese *(Oven Poppers),* 5-oz. piece . . 150

Coffee, instant, regular, 1 rounded tsp.* 4

Coffee, flavored, see "Coffee, iced" and "Cappuccino"

Coffee, flavored, mix, 8 fl. oz.*:

all flavors, except French vanilla *(General Foods
   International* Low Calorie) 30

Belgian hazelnut *(General Foods International)* 70

cafe Amaretto or Français *(General Foods International)* . . 60

cafe Vienna *(General Foods International)* 70

cappuccino, cinnamon, coffee, or vanilla *(Maxwell
   House)*. 90

cappuccino, Italian *(General Foods International)* 50

cappuccino, mocha *(Maxwell House)* 100

French vanilla *(General Foods International)* 60

French vanilla *(General Foods International* Low Calorie) . . 35

Kahlua Cafe or Suisse mocha *(General Foods
   International)* 60

Viennese chocolate *(General Foods International)* 60

Coffee creamer, see "Creamer, nondairy"

Coffee substitute, cereal grain:

(Natural Touch Kaffree Roma), 1 tsp. 10

(Natural Touch Roma Cappuccino), 3 tbsp. 50

(Postum), 1 tsp. 10

Cold cuts, see "Lunch meat" and specific listings

Collard greens, ½ cup:

fresh, raw, chopped 6

fresh, boiled, drained, chopped 17

canned *(Allens/Sunshine)* 30

canned, seasoned *(Sylvia's)* 45

frozen, chopped, boiled, drained 31

Cookie (see also "Cake, snack"):

almond *(Anna's),* 7 pieces, 1 oz. 141

almond *(Stella D'oro* Breakfast Treats), 1 piece, .8 oz. . . . 100

almond *(Stella D'oro* Chinese Dessert), 1 piece, 1.2 oz. . . 170

almond toast *(Stella D'oro* Mandel), 2 pieces, 1 oz. 110

animal, iced or sprinkled *(Keebler),* 6 pieces, 1.1 oz. 150

animal, chocolate chip *(Keebler)*, 7 pieces, 1 oz. 130
anisette *(Stella D'oro* Toast), 3 pieces, 1.2 oz. 130
anisette *(Stella D'oro* Jumbo Toast), 1 piece, 1.1 oz. . . . 100
apple cinnamon *(Newton Cobblers)*, 1 piece, .75 oz. 70
apple filled *(Fig Newton* Fat Free), 2 pieces, 1 oz. 90
biscotti, almond *(Perugina)*, 1 piece 120
biscotti, hazelnut *(Stella D'oro)*, 1 piece, .8 oz. 100
biscottini cashews *(Stella D'oro)*, 1 piece, .7 oz. 110
butter *(Keebler)*, 5 pieces, 1.1 oz. 150
butter *(Keebler Cookie Stix)*, 4 pieces, 1 oz. 130
butter *(Sunshine All American)*, 5 pieces, 1.1 oz. 140
butter sandwich, w/fudge *(E. L. Fudge)*, 2 pieces, .9 oz. . . 120
chocolate *(Stella D'oro* Breakfast Treat), 1 piece, .8 oz. . . 100
chocolate *(Stella D'oro* Castelets), 2 pieces, 1 oz. 130
chocolate wafer *(Nabisco Famous)*, 5 pieces, 1.2 oz. . . . 140
chocolate chip:
   (Chips Ahoy!), 3 pieces, 1.1 oz. 160
   (Chips Ahoy! Chewy), 3 pieces, 1.3 oz. 170
   (Chips Ahoy! Chunky), 1 piece, .6 oz. 80
   (Chips Ahoy! Munch Size), 6 pieces, 1.1 oz. 160
   (Entenmann's Original), 3 pieces, 1.1 oz. 150
   (Grandma's Rich N'Chewy), 1 pkg. 270
   (Keebler Chips Deluxe), 1 piece, .5 oz. 80
   (Keebler Cookie Stix), 4 pieces, 1 oz. 130
   coconut or rainbow *(Keebler Chips Deluxe)*, 1 piece,
     .5 oz. 80
   reduced fat *(Keebler Chips Deluxe)*, 1 piece, .6 oz. 70
   soft *(Keebler Soft Batch)*, 1 piece, .6 oz. 80
chocolate fudge:
   (Grandma's Cookie Bits), 9 pieces 150
   (Keebler Classic Collection), 1 piece, .6 oz. 80
   center *(Health Valley)*, 2 pieces 70
   mint *(Fudge Shoppe* Grasshoppers), 4 pieces,
     1.1 oz. 150
   nutty *(Grandma's* Big), 1 piece, 1.4 oz. 180
   sticks *(Fudge Shoppe)*, 3 pieces, 1 oz. 150
   striped *(Fudge Favorites)*, 3 pieces, 1.1 oz. 160
chocolate sandwich:
   (Hydrox), 3 pieces, 1.1 oz. 150
   (Oreo), 3 pieces, 1.2 oz. 160

Cookie, chocolate sandwich *(cont.)*

   (Oreo Double Stuff), 2 pieces, 1 oz. 140

   (SnackWell's), 2 pieces, .9 oz. 110

   dark, w/vanilla or fudge *(E. L. Fudge)*, 2 pieces,

     .9 oz. 120

   white fudge covered *(Oreo)*, 1 piece, ¾ oz. 110

cinnamon raisin *(Stella D'oro)*, 1 piece, 1 oz. 110

cranberry *(Fig Newton* Fat Free)*, 2 pieces, 1 oz. 100

cranberry *(Golden Fruit* Biscuits)*, 1 piece, .7 oz. 80

creme sandwich *(SnackWell's)*, 2 pieces, .9 oz. 110

Danish *(Keebler* Wedding)*, 4 pieces, 1 oz. 120

date *(Health Valley* Delight)*, 3 pieces 100

devil's food *(SnackWell's)*, 1 piece, .6 oz. 50

egg biscuit *(Stella D'oro* Jumbo)*, 2 pieces, .8 oz. 90

fig filled *(Fig Newton)*, 2 pieces, 1.1 oz. 110

fortune *(Frieda's)*, 4 pieces, 1 oz. 120

fruit, tropical *(Health Valley)*, 3 pieces 100

golden bar *(Stella D'oro)*, 1 piece, 1 oz. 110

ginger lemon creme *(Carr's)*, 2 pieces, 1 oz. 140

ginger snaps *(Nabisco)*, 4 pieces, 1 oz. 120

ginger snaps *(Sunshine)*, 5 pieces, 1.2 oz. 150

graham cracker:

   (Cinnamon Crisps Graham Selects), 8 pieces, 1.1 oz. . 140

   (Graham Selects), 8 pieces, 1 oz. 130

   (Honey Graham Selects), 8 pieces, 1.1 oz. 150

   (Honey Maid), 8 pieces, 1 oz. 120

   (Honey Maid Low Fat)*, 8 pieces, 1 oz. 110

   (Honey Snackin' Grahams Bite Size)*, 23 pieces,

     1.1 oz. 130

   (Nabisco), 4 pieces, 1 oz. 120

   amaranth *(Health Valley* Original)*, 6 pieces 120

   cinnamon *(Honey Maid)*, 8 pieces, 1 oz. 120

   cinnamon *(Honey Maid* Low Fat)*, 8 pieces, 1 oz. . . . 110

   cinnamon *(Sweet Crispers* Snacks)*, 18 pieces,

     1.1 oz. 130

   honey *(Teddy Grahams* Snacks)*, 24 pieces, 1.1 oz. . . 140

   oatmeal crunch *(Honey Maid)*, 8 pieces, 1 oz. 120

graham, chocolate:

   (Fudge Favorites), 3 pieces, 1 oz. 140

   (Fudge Shoppe Deluxe), 3 pieces, .9 oz. 140

(Graham Selects), 8 pieces, 1.1 oz. 130
(Honey Maid), 8 pieces, 1 oz. 120
(Sweet Crispers Snacks), 18 pieces, 1.1 oz. 130
kichel *(Manischewitz)*, 4 pieces, .5 oz. 70
kichel *(Stella D'oro* Low Sodium), 21 pieces, 1 oz. . . . 150
lemon *(Sunshine All American)*, 5 pieces, 1.1 oz. 140
lemon w/hazelnuts *(Larzaroni)*, 5 pieces, 1 oz. 140
marshmallow, chocolate *(Mallomars)*, 2 pieces, .9 oz. . . . 120
mint creme *(SnackWell's)*, 2 pieces, .9 oz. 110
molasses *(Grandma's* Big), 1 piece, 1.4 oz. 160
oatmeal *(Keebler Classic Collection)*, 2 pieces, 1.1 oz. . . . 150
oatmeal *(Nabisco* Family Favorites), 1 piece, .6 oz. 80
oatmeal *(Sunshine* Country), 1 piece, .5 oz. 80
oatmeal, iced *(Nabisco* Family Favorites), 1 piece, .6 oz. . . 80
oatmeal raisin *(Keebler Soft Batch)*, 1 piece, .6 oz. 70
peach-apricot *(Newton Cobblers)*, 1 piece, .75 oz. 70
peanut butter:
    (Keebler Classic Collection), 2 pieces, 1.1 oz. 150
    (Keebler Cookie Stix), 4 pieces; 1 oz. 130
    chip *(SnackWell's* Bite Size), 13 pieces, 1 oz. 120
    w/chocolate chip *(Grandma's* Big), 1 piece, 1.4 oz. . . . 190
peanut butter sandwich *(Grandma's)*, 5 pieces 210
peanut butter sandwich *(Nutter Butter)*, 2 pieces, 1 oz. . . 130
pfeffernusse *(Stella D'oro)*, 3 pieces, 1 oz. 120
praline, chocolate coated *(Bahlsen* Pralinette), 4 pieces,
    1 oz. 150
raisin *(Golden Fruit* Biscuits), 1 piece, .7 oz. 80
raspberry filled *(Fig Newton* Fat Free), 2 pieces, 1 oz. . . . 100
sesame *(Stella D'oro* Regina), 3 pieces, 1.1 oz. 150
shortbread *(Lorna Doone)*, 4 pieces, 1 oz. 140
shortbread *(Pecan Sandies/Almond Sandies)*, 1 piece,
    .6 oz. 80
shortbread *(Sugar Kake)*, 4 pieces, 1 oz. 140
(Social Tea), 6 pieces, 1 oz. 120
(Stella D'oro Lady Stella Assortment), 3 pieces, 1 oz. . . . 130
(Stella D'oro Margherite), 2 pieces, 1.1 oz. 140
sugar *(Keebler Classic Collection)*, 2 pieces, 1 oz. 140
sugar wafer *(Keebler)*, 3 pieces, 1 oz. 150
sugar wafer *(Sunshine)*, 3 pieces, .9 oz. 130
sugar wafer, creme filled *(Biscos)*, 9 pieces, 1 oz. 140

Cookie *(cont.)*

sugar wafer, w/peanut butter *(Sunshine)*, 4 pieces,
   1.1 oz. 170
strawberry filled *(Fig Newton* Fat Free), 2 pieces, 1 oz. . . . 100
vanilla:
   (Grandma's Cookie Bits), 9 pieces 150
   (Keebler Classic Collection), 1 piece, .6 oz. 80
   wafer *(Keebler)*, 8 pieces, 1.1 oz. 150
   wafer, reduced fat *(Keebler)*, 8 pieces, 1.1 oz. 130
   wafer *(Nilla)*, 8 pieces, 1.1 oz. 140
   wafer *(Nilla* Reduced Fat), 8 pieces, 1 oz. 120
   wafer, chocolate *(Nilla* Reduced Fat), 8 pieces, 1 oz. . . 110
vanilla sandwich *(Cameo)*, 2 pieces, 1 oz. 130
vanilla sandwich *(Grandma's)*, 1 pkg. 210
vanilla sandwich *(Vienna Fingers)*, 2 pieces, 1 oz. 140
waffle *(Bahlsen)*, 5 pieces, 1 oz. 160
Cookie, mix*, 2 pieces, except as noted:
chocolate chip or peanut butter *(Betty Crocker)* 160
chocolate chunk, double *(Betty Crocker)* 150
chocolate or espresso chip *(Arrowhead Mills)*, 1 piece 80
oatmeal chocolate chip *(Betty Crocker)* 160
oatmeal raisin *(Arrowhead Mills)*, 1 piece 70
sugar *(Betty Crocker)* 170
Cookie, refrigerated, 1 oz., except as noted:
(Pillsbury M&M's) 130
chocolate, double *(Pillsbury)* 130
chocolate chip *(Nestlé/Nestlé* Big Batch), 2 tbsp. 140
chocolate chip *(Nestlé* Reduced Fat), 2 tbsp. 130
chocolate chip *(Pillsbury)* 130
chocolate chip *(Pillsbury* Reduced Fat) 110
chocolate chip, oatmeal *(Pillsbury)* 120
chocolate chip, peanut butter *(Nestlé)*, 2 tbsp. 160
chocolate chip, w/walnuts *(Pillsbury)* 140
chocolate chunk *(Pillsbury)* 130
holiday shapes *(Pillsbury)* 130
oatmeal *(Nestlé Scotchies)*, 2 tbsp. 140
peanut butter *(Pillsbury)* 120
peanut butter *(Pillsbury Reese's)* 130
sugar *(Nestlé)*, ½" slice 120
sugar *(Pillsbury)* 130

Cookie crumbs, graham *(Honey Maid)*, 2.5 tbsp. 70
Cookie pie crust, see "Pie crust"
Cooking sauce, see specific listings
Coquito nuts *(Frieda's)*, 11 pieces, 1 oz. 110
Coriander:
fresh, ¼ cup 1
dried, leaf, 1 tsp. 2
dried, seed, 1 tsp. 5
Corkscrew pasta dishes, mix, dry:
four-cheese sauce *(DeBoles)*, 2 oz. 220
w/herb-garlic sauce *(Annie's)*, ⅔ cup 260
Corn, fresh, kernels, boiled, drained, ½ cup 89
Corn, canned, ½ cup, except as noted:
kernel, golden:
   (Del Monte) 90
   (Del Monte Supersweet) 60
   (Del Monte Supersweet Vac Pack) 70
   (Green Giant/Green Giant 50% Less Sodium) 80
   (Green Giant Niblets), ⅓ cup 70
   (Green Giant Niblets Extra Sweet), ⅓ cup 50
   (Green Giant Niblets Less Sodium/No Salt/Sugar), ⅓
     cup 60
   (Seneca) 90
   (Seneca No Salt) 80
kernel, golden and white *(Del Monte Supersweet)* 80
kernel, white *(Del Monte)* 60
kernel, white *(Seneca Super Sweet)* 100
kernel, w/peppers *(Del Monte Fiesta)* 50
kernel, w/peppers *(Green Giant Mexicorn)*, ⅓ cup 60
cream style, golden *(Del Monte)* 90
cream style *(Del Monte Supersweet)* 60
cream style *(Green Giant)* 100
cream style *(Seneca)* 80
cream style, white *(Del Monte)* 100
Corn, frozen:
on the cob, 1 ear:
   (Green Giant Extra Sweet) 120
   (Green Giant Niblets) 160
   (Green Giant Nibblers) 70
   (John Cope's) 140

Corn, frozen, on the cob *(cont.)*

(*John Cope's* Mini) 80
(*Seneca*) 140
kernel:
(*Cascadian Farm*), ³/₄ cup 90
(*Green Giant Niblets*), ²/₃ cup 80
(*Green Giant Niblets* Extra Sweet), ²/₃ cup 70
(*Green Giant Niblets Harvest Fresh*), ²/₃ cup 80
(*John Cope's* Shoepeg), ²/₃ cup 80
(*Seneca*), ²/₃ cup 90
white (*Green Giant* Select Extra Sweet), ²/₃ cup 50
white (*Green Giant* Select Shoepeg), ³/₄ cup 100
white (*Green Giant Harvest Fresh* Shoepeg), ¹/₂ cup . . . 70
creamed (*Seabrook*), ¹/₂ cup 170
in butter sauce (*Cascadian Farm*), ¹/₂ cup 100
in butter sauce (*Green Giant Niblets*), ²/₃ cup 130
in butter sauce, white (*Green Giant*), ³/₄ cup 120
cream style (*Green Giant*), ¹/₂ cup 110
seasoned (*Green Giant* Southwestern), ³/₄ cup 90
Corn, dried (*Frieda's* Posole), ¹/₃ cup 30
Corn bran, crude, ¹/₄ cup 43
Corn bread, mix*:
(*Ballard*), ¹/₁₈ loaf 130
buttermilk (*Martha White*), ¹/₅ pan 140
buttermilk (*Martha White Cotton Pickin*), ¹/₅ pan 170
chili (*Martha White* Fiesta), ¹/₆ pan 190
honey, golden (*Martha White*), ¹/₆ pan 170
Mexican (*Gladiola*), ¹/₆ pan 130
Mexican (*Martha White*), ¹/₆ pan 140
yellow (*Martha White*), ¹/₅ pan 160
yellow or white (*Gladiola*), ¹/₆ pan 140
white (*Burrus Light Crust*), ¹/₆ pan 140
Corn bread, refrigerated, twists (*Pillsbury*), 1 piece 140
Corn chips, puffs, and similar snacks (see also "Snack
chips and crisps"), 1 oz., except as noted:
(*Baked Bugles*), 1.1 oz. 130
(*Bugles*), 1.1 oz. 160
(*Dipsy Doodles*) 160
(*Fritos/Fritos* King Size/Scoops) 160
(*Frito-Lay Funyons*) 140

(Frito-Lay Munchos) 160
barbecue *(Bugels* Smokin), 1.1 oz. 150
barbecue *(Fritos)* 150
barbecue *(Frito-Lay Munchos)* 160
barbecue *(Wise)* 150
barbecue, honey *(Fritos* Texas Grill) 150
barbecue, mesquite *(Dipsy Doodles)* 160
caramel puffs *(Health Valley)*, 2 cups 120
cheese:
   (Chee•tos Checkers/Crunchy/Puffs) 160
   (Chee•tos Curls/Puffed Balls) 150
   cheddar *(Baked Bugels)*, 1.1 oz. 130
   cheddar *(Dipsy Doodles)* 150
   cheddar *(Dipsy Doodles* Reduced Fat) 130
   cheddar *(Wise* Baked Puffed Balls) 140
   cheddar *(Wise* Baked Puffs) 150
   cheddar *(Wise* Puffed Doodles) 120
   chili *(Fritos)* 160
   hot *(Chee•tos* Flamin') 160
   nacho *(Bugels)*, 1.1 oz. 160
   nacho *(Chee•tos)* 160
   pizza *(Wise Crunchers)* 160
hot *(Sabrositas* Flamin') 150
lime and chili *(Sabrositas)* 150
ranch *(Fritos* Wild 'N Mild) 160
sour cream and onion *(Bugels)*, 1.1 oz. 160
tortilla:
   (Moore's Tostado Rounds) 150
   (Santitas Chips/Strips) 140
   (Tostitos Baked) 110
   (Tostitos Bite Size/Restaurant/Santa Fe Gold) 140
   (Tostitos Crispy Rounds) 150
   (Tyson Salted) 150
   all varieties *(Doritos)* 140
   all varieties *(Valley of Mexico)* 140
   all varieties *(Wise)* 150
   cheese and salsa *(Tostitos)* 140
   lime and chili *(Tostitos)* 150
   nacho cheese *(Doritos* Cheesier/Spicy/3D's Cheesier) . 140
   nacho cheese *(Tostitos)* 140

Corn chips, puffs, and similar snacks, tortilla *(cont.)*
nacho cheese *(Wise Bravo)* 150
nacho cheese, reduced fat *(Doritos Wow!)* 90
salsa and sour cream *(Tostitos Baked)* 120
taco *(Taco Bell Supreme)* 150
white corn *(Santitas)* 140
yellow *(Tyson)* 150
Corn flake crumbs, see "Cereal crumbs"
Corn flour:
whole-grain, 1 cup 422
masa, 1 cup 416
Corn grits, dry, ¼ cup, except as noted:
(Albers) 140
(Jim Dandy) 170
(Jim Dandy Quick) 160
(Jim Dandy Quick Iron Fortified) 140
(Martha White Instant), 1 oz. 100
bacon *(Martha White Instant)*, 1 oz. 110
white *(Arrowhead Mills)* 140
yellow *(Arrowhead Mills)* 130
yellow *(Martha White)* 150
Corn relish *(Green Giant)*, 1 tbsp. 20
Corn soufflé, frozen *(Stouffer's Side Dish)*, ½ cup . . . 170
Cornish hen, raw, frozen *(Tyson)*, 4 oz. 180
Cornmeal (see also "Corn flour" and "Polenta"):
blue *(Arrowhead Mills)*, ¼ cup 130
buttermilk mix *(Gladiola/Martha White Self-Rising)*,
   3 tbsp. 110
white *(Jim Dandy)*, 3 tbsp. 120
white *(Jim Dandy Self-Rising)*, 3 tbsp. 110
white *(Martha White/Hay Market)*, 3 tbsp. 120
white or yellow *(Albers)*, 3 tbsp. 110
whole ground *(Cabin Home)*, 3 tbsp. 110
whole ground *(Cabin Home Self-Rising)*, 3 tbsp. 110
yellow *(Arrowhead Mills)*, ¼ cup 120
yellow, *(Martha White)*, 3 tbsp. 120
yellow, mix *(Martha White Self-Rising)*, 3 tbsp. 110
Cornstarch *(Argo/Kingsford)*, 1 tbsp. 30
Cottonseed kernels, roasted, 1 tbsp. 51
Cottonseed meal, partially defatted, 1 oz. 104

Country gravy, mix *(Loma Linda Gravy Quik)*, 1 tbsp. 25
Couscous:
dry *(Arrowhead Mills)*, ¼ cup 170
dry, regular or whole wheat *(Fantastic Foods)*, ¼ cup . . . 210
cooked, ½ cup 101
Couscous dishes, mix, dry. 1 pkg., except as noted:
black bean salsa *(Fantastic Foods Cup)* 240
cheddar, nacho *(Fantastic Foods Cup)* 200
corn, sweet *(Fantastic Foods Cup)* 180
Creole vegetable *(Fantastic Foods Cup)* 220
garlic, w/red pepper *(Fantastic Foods Healthy*
    Complements), ⅓ cup 200
lentil curry *(Marrakesh Express)*, ½ cup* 130
Thai, royal *(Fantastic Foods Healthy Complements)*,
    ⅓ cup 200
Cowpeas, ½ cup, except as noted:
fresh, boiled, drained 79
fresh, leafy tips, boiled, drained, 4 oz. 25
fresh, pods, w/seeds, boiled, drained 16
canned, see "Black-eye peas"
frozen, boiled, drained 112
Crab, meat only, 4 oz.:
Alaska king, raw 95
Alaska king, boiled, poached, or steamed 110
blue, raw 99
blue, boiled, poached, or steamed 116
Dungeness, raw 98
Dungeness, boiled, poached, or steamed 125
queen, raw 102
queen, boiled, poached, or steamed 130
Crab, canned, blue, 4 oz. 112
Crab, frozen:
cakes *(Van de Kamp's)*, 1 piece 170
cakes, deviled *(Mrs. Paul's)*, 1 piece 170
cakes, mini *(Mrs. Paul's)*, 6 pieces 230
"Crab," imitation, frozen or refrigerated:
chunk or flakes *(Louis Kemp Crab Delights)*, ½ cup 90
flakes *(Captain Jac Crab Tasties)*, ½ cup 100
flakes *(Seafest)*, ½ cup 100
leg style *(Captain Jac Crab Tasties)*, 3 legs, 3 oz. 90

74 *Corinne T. Netzer*

"Crab," imitation *(cont.)*
leg style *(Louis Kemp Crab Delights)*, 3 legs, 3 oz. 90
leg style *(Seafest)*, 3 legs, 3 oz. 90
Crabapple, fresh, sliced, ½ cup 42
Crab cake, see "Crab, frozen"
Cracker:
almond *(Blue Diamond Nut Thins)*, 16 pieces, 1.1 oz. . . . 130
arrowroot *(Nabisco)*, 1 piece, .2 oz. 20
butter *(Hi-Ho)*, 4 pieces, .5 oz. 70
butter *(Hi-Ho Reduced Fat)*, 5 pieces, .5 oz. 70
butter *(Keebler Club)*, 4 pieces, .5 oz. 70
butter *(Ritz Air Crisps)*, 24 pieces 140
butter *(Ritz Original/Low Sodium)*, 5 pieces, .6 oz. 80
butter *(Town House)*, 5 pieces, .6 oz. 80
butter *(Town House Reduced Fat)*, 6 pieces, .5 oz. 70
butter crisp *(Toasteds)*, 5 pieces, .6 oz. 80
cheese:
    (BIG Cheez-It), 13 pieces, 1 oz. 150
    (Cheez-It), 27 pieces, 1.1 oz. 160
    (Cheez-It Low Fat), 29 pieces, 1.1 oz. 140
    (Cheez-It Low Sodium), 27 pieces, 1.1 oz. 160
    (Cheese Nips), 29 pieces, 1.1 oz. 150
    (Cheese Nips Air Crisps), 32 pieces, 1.1 oz. 130
    (Tid-Bit), 32 pieces 160
    cheddar *(Better Cheddars)*, 22 pieces, 1.1 oz. 150
    cheddar *(Better Cheddars Lowfat)*, 24 pieces, 1.1 oz. . 140
    cheddar *(Krispy)*, 5 pieces, .5 oz. 60
    cheddar *(Munch 'ems)*, 30 pieces, 1.1 oz. 130
    cheddar, white *(Cheez-It)*, 26 pieces, 1.1 oz. 150
    hot, spicy *(Cheez-It)*, 26 pieces, 1.1 oz. 160
    nacho *(Cheez-It)*, 28 pieces, 1.1 oz. 150
    and sesame *(Twigs)*, 15 pieces 150
    Swiss *(Nabisco)*, 15 pieces 140
cheese sandwich:
    (Handi-Snacks), 1.1-oz. pkg. 130
    (Ritz Bits), 14 pieces 170
    cheddar *(Frito-Lay)*, 1 pkg. 200
    cheddar *(Keebler Club)*, 1 pkg., 1.3 oz. 190
    cheesy *(Chee•tos)*, 1 pkg. 210
    w/bacon *(Chee•tos)*, 1 pkg. 190

nacho *(Doritos* Cheesier), 1 pkg. 240
w/peanut butter *(Keebler),* 1 pkg., 1.3 oz. 190
w/peanut butter *(Peter Pan* Cheese), 1 pkg. 210
spicy *(Doritos),* 1 pkg. 230
(Chicken In A Biscuit), 12 pieces 160
garlic, roasted *(Health Valley* Low Fat), 6 pieces 60
graham crackers, see "Cookies"
herb, garden *(Triscuit),* 6 pieces, 1 oz. 130
herb, Italian *(Harvest Crisp),* 13 pieces 130
herb, whole wheat *(Health Valley),* 5 pieces 50
jalapeño, mild *(Health Valley* Low Fat), 6 pieces 60
matzo:
    (Manischewitz Everything!), 12 pieces, 1 oz. 110
    garlic *(Manischewitz),* 12 pieces, 1 oz. 100
    Passover *(Manischewitz* Tam Tam), 10 pieces,
      1.1 oz. 140
    thins *(Manischewitz),* 1 piece, .8 oz. 90
    unsalted *(Manischewitz),* 1 piece, 1 oz. 110
multigrain *(Harvest Crisp),* 13 pieces, 1.1 oz. 130
multi-grain *(Saltines),* 5 pieces, .5 oz. 60
(Munch 'ems), 35 pieces, 1.1 oz. 130
oat bran *(Health Valley),* 6 pieces 120
onion *(Toasteds),* 5 pieces, .6 oz. 80
onion, French *(SnackWell's),* 38 pieces 130
onion, French *(Triscuit* Thin Crisps), 14 pieces, 1.1 oz. . . 130
peanut butter sandwich, see also "cheese sandwich,"
  above
    (Ritz Bits), 14 pieces 150
    toast *(Keebler),* 1 pkg. 190
    toast *(Keebler* Reduced Fat), 1 pkg. 170
pecan *(Blue Diamond* Nut Thins), 16 pieces, 1.1 oz. 130
pizza, all varieties *(Health Valley* Healthy Pizza), 6 pieces . . 50
potato, barbecue *(Air Crisps),* 22 pieces, 1 oz. 120
potato, ranch *(Air Crisps),* 23 pieces, 1.1 oz. 140
pretzel *(Air Crisps),* 23 pieces 110
ranch *(Munch 'ems),* 33 pieces, 1.1 oz. 130
ranch *(Wheatables),* 25 pieces, 1.1 oz. 150
salsa *(Munch 'ems* Southwest), 28 pieces, 1.1 oz. 130
saltines, 5 pieces, .5 oz.:
    (Krispy Fat Free) 50

Cracker, saltines *(cont.)*
   (Krispy/Krispy Unsalted) 60
   (Zesta) 60
   (Zesta Fat Free) 50
   (Zesta Low Salt/Unsalted) 70
   all varieties *(Saltines)* 60
sandwich *(Chee•tos* Golden Toast), 1 pkg. 240
sesame *(Toasteds)*, 5 pieces, .6 oz. 80
sesame *(Toasteds* Reduced Fat), 5 pieces, .5 oz. 60
(Sociables), 7 pieces, .5 oz. 80
soda/water *(Crown Pilot)*, 1 piece, .6 oz. 70
soda/water *(Export)*, 3 pieces, .5 oz. 60
soda/water *(Royal Lunch)*, 1 piece, .4 oz. 60
soda/water cracked pepper *(SnackWell's)*, 5 pieces,
   .5 oz. 60
soup and oyster *(Zesta)*, 45 pieces, .5 oz. 70
sour cream-onion *(Munch 'ems)*, 28 pieces, 1.1 oz. . . . 140
sour cream-onion *(Ritz* Air Crisps), 23 pieces, 1.1 oz. . . 140
(Uneeda Biscuit), 2 pieces, .5 oz. 60
vegetable *(Nabisco Thins)*, 14 pieces 160
vegetable, garden *(Harvest Crisp)*, 15 pieces 130
vegetable, garden *(Wheatables)*, 25 pieces 140
wheat:
   (SnackWell's), 5 pieces, .5 oz. 70
   (Toasteds), 5 pieces, .6 oz. 80
   (Toasteds Reduced Fat), 5 pieces, .5 oz. 60
   (Triscuit Original/Low Sodium), 7 pieces, 1.1 oz. 140
   (Triscuit Reduced Fat), 8 pieces, 1.2 oz. 130
   (Triscuit Thin Crisps), 15 pieces, 1.1 oz. 130
   (Waverly), 5 pieces, .5 oz. 70
   (Wheatables), 26 pieces, 1.1 oz. 150
   (Wheatables Reduced Fat), 27 pieces, 1.1 oz. 130
   (Wheat Thins Air Crisps), 24 pieces, 1.1 oz. 130
   (Wheat Thins Big), 11 pieces, 1.1 oz. 140
   (Wheat Thins Multi-grain), 17 pieces, 1.1 oz. 130
   (Wheat Thins Original), 16 pieces, .8 oz. 140
   (Wheat Thins Reduced Fat), 18 pieces 120
   (Wheatsworth), 5 pieces, .6 oz. 80
   whole *(Hi-Ho)*, 4 pieces, .5 oz. 70
   whole *(Krispy)*, 5 pieces, .5 oz. 60

zweiback *(Nabisco)*, 1 piece, .3 oz. 35
Cracker crumbs and meal:
crumbs *(Ritz)*, ⅓ cup 140
crumbs, graham cracker *(Sunshine)*, 3 tbsp. 80
crumbs, saltine *(Premium* Fat Free), ¼ cup 100
meal *(Nabisco)*, ¼ cup 110
meal, matzo *(Manischewitz)*, ¼ cup 130
Cranberry, fresh:
(Ocean Spray), 2 oz. 25
chopped, ½ cup 27
Cranberry, dried *(Craisins)*, ⅓ cup 130
Cranberry bean:
boiled, ½ cup 120
canned, ½ cup 108
Cranberry drink, 8 fl. oz.:
juice cocktail *(Ocean Spray)* 140
juice cocktail *(Ocean Spray Lightstyle)* 40
juice cocktail, reduced calorie *(Ocean Spray)* 50
Cranberry drink blends, 8 fl. oz., except as noted:
apple *(Cranapple)* 160
apple *(Tropicana Twister)* 140
apricot *(Cranicot)* 160
(Cran•Blueberry/Cran•Cherry) 160
(Cran•Currant) 140
grape *(Cran•Grape)* 170
grape *(Cran•Grape Lightstyle)* 40
mango *(Cran•Mango)* 130
mango *(Cran•Mango Lightstyle)* 40
punch *(Tropicana Twister)*, 10 fl. oz. 170
raspberry *(Cran•Raspberry)* 140
raspberry *(Cran•Raspberry Lightstyle)* 40
strawberry *(Cran•Strawberry)* 140
strawberry *(Tropicana Twister)* 120
strawberry *(Tropicana Twister* Light) 35
strawberry, reduced calorie *(Cran•Raspberry)* 50
tangerine *(Cran•Tangerine)* 130
Cranberry juice, 8 fl. oz.:
(Season's Best Cocktail) 140
(Wellfleet Farms) 130

Cranberry juice blend, 8 fl. oz.:
(Season's Best Medley) 120
apple *(Dole)* 120
apple, Granny Smith *(Wellfleet Farms)* 130
lime, key *(Wellfleet Farms)* 140
peach, Georgia *(Wellfleet Farms)* 140
Cranberry sauce, canned, whole or jellied
(Ocean Spray), ¼ cup 110
Cranberry sauce blends, w/orange, raspberry, or
  strawberry *(Cran•Fruit),* ¼ cup 120
Cranberry-orange relish, in jars *(New England),* ¼ cup . 120
Crayfish, mixed species, meat only:
farmed, raw, 4 oz. 82
farmed, boiled or steamed, 4 oz. 99
wild, raw, 4 oz. 87
wild, raw, 8 medium, 1 oz. 22
wild, boiled or steamed, 4 oz. 100
Cream (see also "Crème fraîche"):
half and half, 1 tbsp. 20
light, coffee, or table, 1 tbsp. 29
medium (25% fat), 1 tbsp. 37
sour, see "Cream, sour"
whipped topping, see "Cream topping"
whipping (volume is doubled when whipped):
  light, 1 cup 699
  light, 1 tbsp. 44
  heavy, 1 cup 821
  heavy, 1 tbsp. 52
Cream, sour, 2 tbsp.:
(Breakstone's) 60
(Friendship) 60
half and half *(Breakstone's)* 45
light *(Friendship)* 40
light *(Hood)* 35
nonfat *(Breakstone's Free/Sealtest Free)* 35
nonfat *(Friendship)* 25
Cream, sour, flavored, 2 tbsp.:
roasted garlic *(Friendship)* 60
salsa *(Friendship)* 60
Cream of tartar *(Tone's),* 1 tsp. 2

Cream topping, 2 tbsp.:
(Cool Whip Extra Creamy) 30
(Cool Whip Lite) 20
(Cool Whip Nondairy) 25
(Kraft Real/Whipped) 20
(La Crema Lite) 15
mix* *(D-Zerta)* 10
Creamer, nondairy:
(Coffee-mate), 1 tbsp. 20
(Hood), 1 tbsp. 20
(Rich's Coffee Rich), 1 tbsp. 25
(Rich's Coffee Rich Light), 1 tbsp. 15
flavored, all flavors *(Coffee-mate),* 1 tbsp. 40
dry *(Coffee-mate/Coffee-mate* Lite), 1 tsp. 10
dry *(Cremora/Cremora* Fat Free/Lite), 1 tsp. 10
dry, flavored, all flavors *(Coffee-mate),* 1⅓ tbsp. 60
Crème fraîche *(Santè)*, 2 tbsp. 100
Cress, garden (see also "Watercress"), raw, ½ cup 8
Croaker, meat only, raw, Atlantic, 4 oz. 119
Croissant, 1 piece:
butter *(Awrey's),* 1½ oz. 140
butter *(Awrey's),* 2 oz. 190
dill and onion or pesto Parmesan *(Awrey's),* 2½ oz. 210
margarine *(Awrey's* Sandwich), 1.8 oz. 180
margarine *(Awrey's Sandwich),* 2½ oz. 250
Croissant, frozen:
French style *(Sara Lee),* 1 piece 170
French style, petite *(Sara Lee),* 2 pieces 230
Crookneck squash:
fresh, sliced, boiled, drained, ½ cup 18
canned, cut, drained, ½ cup 14
frozen, boiled, sliced, sliced, ½ cup 24
Croutons (see also "Salad toppers"), ¼ oz. or 2 tbsp.:
all varieties *(Arnold* Crispy/*Brownberry)* 30
all varieties *(Old London* Restaurant Style) 30
Caesar *(Pepperidge Farm)* 35
cheddar and Romano *(Pepperidge Farm)* 30
cheese and garlic *(Pepperidge Farm)* 35
seasoned *(Pepperidge Farm)* 35
Cruller, see "Donut"

Cucumber, w/peel:
1 medium, 8¼″ long 38
sliced, ½ cup 7
Japanese or hothouse *(Frieda's)*, ⅔ cup, 3 oz. 10
Cucumber, pickled, see "Pickles"
Cucumber dip, creamy *(Kraft* Premium), 2 tbsp. 50
Cuczza squash *(Frieda's)*, ¾ cup, 3 oz. 10
Cumin seed, ground, 1 tsp. 8
Currant, ½ cup:
fresh, black, Europe 36
fresh, red or white 31
dried, zante 204
Curry paste *(Patak's)*, 2 tbsp. 170
Curry powder, 1 tbsp. 20
Curry sauce, Thai, green *(Ka•Me)*, 1 tbsp. 10
Curry sauce, cooking:
hot, Madras *(Patak's)*, ½ cup 300
hot, tikka Masala *(Patak's)*, ½ cup 240
hot, vindaloo *(Patak's)*, ½ cup 320
Jalfrezzi *(Patak's)*, ½ cup 160
Masala *(Shahi* Cream/Curry), ¼ cup 50
rogan josh *(Patak's)*, ½ cup 190
Cusk, meat only:
raw, 4 oz. 99
baked, broiled, or microwaved, 4 oz. 127
Custard, see "Pudding mix"
Custard apple, trimmed, 1 oz. 29
Cuttlefish, meat only:
raw, 4 oz. 90
boiled or steamed, 4 oz. 179
Cuttlefish, canned, in ink *(Goya)*, ¼ cup 120

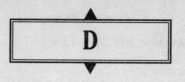

D

FOOD AND MEASURE   **CALORIES**

Daikon, see "Radish, Oriental"
Daiquiri mixer, Hawaiian *(Trader Vic's),* 4 fl. oz. 170
Dandelion greens:
raw, ½ cup chopped, 1 oz. 13
boiled, drained, chopped, ½ cup 17
Danish, 1 piece:
all varieties *(Awrey's* Petite), 1½ oz. 130
all varieties, except cinnamon roll *(Awrey's),* 2¾ oz. 300
apple *(Awrey's* Grande), 4½ oz. 450
cheese *(Awrey's* Grande), 4½ oz. 480
cherry cheese *(Awrey's* Marquise), 3¼ oz. 350
cinnamon *(Awrey's* Marquise), 4½ oz. 470
cinnamon roll *(Awrey's* Homestyle), 2¾ oz. 270
cinnamon swirl *(Awrey's* Grande), 3¾ oz. 420
lemon cheese *(Awrey's* Marquise), 3¼ oz. 350
raspberry cheese swirl *(Awrey's* Grande), 3¾ oz. 400
strawberry *(Awrey's* Grande), 4½ oz. 480
Danish cake, see "Cake"
Dairy Queen/Brazier, 1 serving:
burgers:
   DQ Homestyle, cheeseburger 340
   DQ Homestyle, cheeseburger, double 540
   DQ Homestyle, cheeseburger, double, w/bacon 610
   DQ Homestyle, hamburger 290
   DQ Ultimate burger 670
sandwiches:
   chicken, grilled 310
   chicken breast fillet 430
   chili 'n' cheese dog 330
   hot dog 240
chicken strip basket 1000
side dishes:
   fries, medium 350
   fries, large 440

Dairy Queen/Brazier, side dishes *(cont.)*

onion rings	320

desserts and shakes:

banana split	510
Blizzard:	
chocolate chip cookie dough, small	660
chocolate chip cookie dough, medium	950
chocolate sandwich cookie, small	520
chocolate sandwich cookie, medium	640
Breeze yogurt, *Heath,* small	470
Breeze yogurt, *Heath,* medium	710
Breeze yogurt, strawberry, small	320
Breeze yogurt, strawberry, medium	460
Buster Bar	450
Chocolate Dilly	210
cone, chocolate, *DQ* soft serve, ½ cup	150
cone, chocolate, small	240
cone, chocolate, medium	340
cone, dipped, small	340
cone, dipped, medium	480
cone, vanilla, *DQ* soft serve, ½ cup	140
cone, vanilla, small	230
cone, vanilla, medium	330
DQ frozen 8″ cake, ⅛ cake	340
DQ fudge bar	50
DQ sandwich	150
DQ Treatzza Pizza, Heath, ⅛ pizza	180
DQ Treatzza Pizza, M&M's, ⅛ pizza	190
DQ vanilla orange bar	60
Fudge Cake Supreme	890
lemon *DQ Freez'r,* ½ cup	80
malt, chocolate, small	650
malt, chocolate, medium	880
Misty slush, small	220
Misty slush, medium	290
Peanut Buster parfait	730
shake, chocolate, small	560
shake, chocolate, medium	770
Starkiss	80
strawberry shortcake	430

sundae, chocolate, small 280
sundae, chocolate, medium 400
yogurt, frozen, cone, medium 260
yogurt, frozen, cup, medium 230
yogurt, frozen, *DQ* nonfat, ½ cup 100
yogurt, frozen, strawberry sundae, medium 280
Date, dried, pitted, natural, dry, 10 dates, 2.9 oz. 228
Date nut loaf, see "Bread, sweet"
Delicata squash *(Frieda's)*, ¾ cup, 3 oz. 30
Dessert, see specific listings
Dessert bar mix, see "Cake, snack, mix"
Diable sauce *(Escoffier)*, 1 tbsp. 20
Dill dip, 2 tbsp.:
(Heluva Good) 60
w/hummus *(Heluva* Good) 50
Dill seed, 1 tsp. 6
Dill weed:
fresh, 5 sprigs . . . . <1
fresh, ½ cup loose packed 2
dried, 1 tsp. 3
Dipping sauce, see specific listings
Dock, boiled, drained, 4 oz. 23
Dolphin fish, meat only:
raw, 4 oz. 97
baked, broiled or microwaved, 4 oz. 124
Domino's Pizza:
medium, 12″, cheese, 2 of 8 slices, except as noted:
  deep dish 477
  hand-tossed 347
  thin crust, ¼ pie 271
  "Add a Topping":
    anchovies 23
    bacon 82
    beef or Italian sausage 55
    cheddar 57
    cheese, extra 48
    ham 17
    mushrooms or onions 4
    olives, green 12
    olives, ripe 14

Domino's Pizza, medium *(cont.)*

onion 4
pepper, green 3
pepperoni 75
pineapple 10

large, 14", cheese, 2 of 12 slices, except as noted:
  deep dish 456
  hand-tossed 317
  thin crust, 1/6 pie 253
  "Add a Topping":
    anchovies 23
    bacon 75
    beef, Italian sausage, or extra cheese 44
    cheddar 48
    ham 17
    mushroom, onion, or banana pepper 3
    olives, green 11
    olives, ripe 12
    pepper, green 2
    pepperoni 66
    pineapple 8

6" deep dish, cheese, 1 pie 595
  "Add a Topping":
    anchovies 45
    bacon 82
    beef or Italian sausage 44
    cheddar 86
    cheese, extra 57
    ham 17
    mushroom or green pepper 2
    olives, green 10
    olives, ripe 11
    onion or banana pepper 3
    pepperoni 49
    pineapple 5

Buffalo wings, barbecue, 1 piece 50
Buffalo wings, hot, 1 piece 45
garden salad, w/out dressing, small 22
garden salad, w/out dressing, large 39

Marzetti salad dressings, 1.5 oz.:

- blue cheese or house Italian 220
- Caesar, creamy, or Thousand Island 200
- honey French 210
- Italian, light 20
- ranch 260
- ranch, fat free 40

breadstick, 1 piece 78
cheesy bread, 1 piece 103

Donut, 1 piece, except as noted:

plain:

- *(Awrey's)*, 1½ oz. 170
- *(Awrey's)*, 2 oz. 240
- *(Entenmann's* Dippers) 160
- *(Entenmann's Popettes)*, 4 pieces 270

blueberry, glazed *(Krispy Kreme)* 300
blueberry filled, powdered *(Krispy Kreme)* 200
cake *(Krispy Kreme* Traditional) 200
cake, chocolate iced *(Entenmann's)* 280
cake, chocolate iced *(Krispy Kreme)* 230
cake, chocolate iced, mini *(Entenmann's)* 150
cake, crumb-topped *(Entenmann's)* 260
cake, milk-chocolate iced *(Entenmann's)* 320
cake, powdered *(Krispy Kreme)* 220

chocolate iced:

- *(Awrey's)*, 2½ oz. 300
- *(Awrey's* Ring), 3 oz. 350
- *(Krispy Kreme)* 260
- chocolate *(Awrey's)*, 1¾ oz. 190
- chocolate *(Awrey's)*, 2½ oz. 280
- creme filled *(Krispy Kreme)* 270
- custard *(Awrey's* Bismark) 350
- custard *(Krispy Kreme)* 250
- sour cream *(Awrey's)* 430
- w/sprinkles *(Krispy Kreme)* 220

cinnamon apple filled *(Krispy Kreme)* 210
coconut top *(Awrey's)* 210
creme filled, glazed *(Krispy Kreme)* 270
cruller *(Entenmann's)* 220
cruller, chocolate iced *(Krispy Kreme)* 240

Donut *(cont.)*
cruller, glazed *(Krispy Kreme)* 220
crunch *(Awrey's)*, 2½ oz. 280
crunch top *(Awrey's)*, 1¾ oz. 160
devil's food *(Entenmann's)* 310
devil's food, glazed *(Krispy Kreme)* 240
devil's food, honey glazed *(Awrey's)* 310
glazed *(Entenmann's Popems)*, 4 pieces 210
glazed *(Krispy Kreme* Original) 170
glazed, honey *(Awrey's* Ring) 310
glazed, stick *(Awrey's* Twin Pack), 2¾ oz. 330
jelly, powdered sugar *(Awrey's* Bismark) 320
lemon-filled *(Krispy Kreme)* 210
maple iced *(Krispy Kreme)* 200
powdered sugar *(Awrey's)*, 1½ oz. 170
powdered sugar *(Awrey's)*, 2¼ oz. 390
raspberry filled *(Krispy Kreme)* 210
sour cream *(Awrey's)* 370
sprinkle top *(Awrey's)* 160
vanilla iced *(Awrey's* Bismark) 320
vanilla iced *(Awrey's* Long John) 380
white iced *(Awrey's)* 200
Donut mix, dry *(Manischewitz Passover Gold)*, ¾ cup . . 270
Dressing, see "Salad dressing" and specific listings
Drum, freshwater, meat only:
raw, 4 oz. 135
baked, broiled, or microwaved, 4 oz. 173
Duck, domesticated, roasted:
meat w/skin, 4 oz. 382
meat only, 4 oz. 228
Duck, wild, raw:
meat w/skin, 4 oz. 239
breast meat, 4 oz. 139
Duck sauce, see "Sweet and sour sauce"
Dumpling entree, Oriental, frozen *(Lean Cuisine)*, 9 oz. . 300

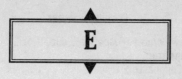

FOOD AND MEASURE   **CALORIES**

Eclair, 1 piece:
chocolate *(Entenmann's)* 260
chocolate, frozen *(Rich's)* 190
Eel, meat only:
raw, 4 oz. 209
baked, broiled, or microwaved, 4 oz. 268
Egg, chicken, 1 large, except as noted:
raw, whole 75
raw, white only 17
raw, yolk only, w/small portion of white 59
cooked, hard-boiled, chopped, 1 cup 210
Egg, substitute, ¼ cup:
(Morningstar Farms Better'n Eggs) 20
(Morningstar Scramblers) 35
Egg, quail, 1 egg 14
Egg pocket, w/sausage, cheese *(Croissant Pockets),*
    4.5 oz. 340
Egg roll, frozen:
chicken *(Chun King* Restaurant Style), 3-oz. roll 190
chicken or pork and shrimp, mini *(Chun King),* 6 rolls . 210
shrimp *(Chun King* Restaurant Style), 3-oz. roll 180
shrimp, mini *(Chun King),* 6 rolls 190
vegetarian *(Worthington),* 1 roll 180
Egg roll entree, frozen, vegetable *(Lean Cuisine),* 9 oz. . 340
Egg roll wrapper:
(Frieda's), 2 130
(Nasoya), 1.5 oz. 117
Eggnog, dairy, ½ cup, except as noted:
(Hood Golden) 180
low fat *(Hood* Light) 140
nonfat *(Hood* Free), 1 cup 110
vanilla *(Hood)* 180
Eggplant, fresh:
boiled, drained, 1″ cubes, ½ cup 13

Japanese, raw, w/peel *(Frieda's)*, ²/₃ cup, 3 oz. 20
Eggplant appetizer:
(Progresso Caponata), 2 tbsp. 25
babaganoush *(Sabra)*, 1 oz. 77
salad, grilled, chopped *(Sabra)*, 1 oz. 61
sliced, Spanish *(Sabra)*, 1 oz. 70
w/tomato *(Sabra* Matbucha Salad), 1 oz. 18
Eggplant pickle relish *(Patak's* Brinjal), 1 tbsp. 60
Elderberry, ¹/₂ cup 53
Enchilada dinner, frozen, 1 pkg.:
beef *(Banquet Extra Helping)*, 15.65 oz. 610
beef *(Patio)*, 12 oz. 370
beef *(Patio* Chili 'N Beans), 15.5 oz. 540
beef and cheese *(Patio* Chili 'N Beans), 15.5 oz. 610
black bean *(Amy's)*, 10 oz. 250
cheese *(Amy's)*, 9 oz. 330
cheese *(Patio)*, 12 oz. 370
chicken *(Healthy Choice* Suprema), 11.3 oz. 300
chicken *(Patio)*, 12 oz. 400
Enchilada entree, frozen, 1 pkg., except as noted:
beef *(Banquet* Meal), 11 oz. 370
beef *(Patio* Family), 2 w/sauce 210
beef and tamale *(Banquet* Meal), 11 oz. 400
black bean vegetable *(Amy's)*, 4³/₄ oz. 130
black bean vegetable *(Amy's* Family Size), 4.38 oz. 120
cheese *(Amy's)*, 4³/₄ oz. 210
cheese *(Amy's* Family Size), 5 oz. 240
cheese *(Banquet* Meal), 11 oz. 360
cheese *(Patio* Family), 2 w/sauce 210
chicken *(Banquet* Meal), 11 oz. 350
chicken *(Stouffer's)*, ¹/₁₂ of 58-oz. pkg. 220
chicken Suiza *(Healthy Choice)*, 10 oz. 280
chicken Suiza, w/Mexican rice *(Lean Cuisine)*, 9 oz. 280
combo *(Banquet* Meal), 11 oz. 360
Enchilada sauce, all varieties *(Old El Paso)*, ¹/₄ cup 30
Enchilada sauce mix *(Old El Paso)*, 2 tsp. 10
Endive, chopped, ¹/₂ cup 4
Endive, Belgian, see "Chicory, witloof"
Escarole, see "Endive"

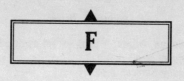

F

FOOD AND MEASURE   **CALORIES**

Fajita dinner mix *(Old El Paso Kit)*, 2 pieces 300
Fajita entree, see "Chicken entree, frozen"
Fajita pocket, frozen, 4.5-oz. piece:
beef *(Hot Pockets)* 340
chicken *(Lean Pockets)* 270
Fajita sauce *(World Harbors Guadalupe Mountain)*,
   2 tbsp. 45
Fajita seasoning *(El Rio)*, 1 tbsp. 5
Fajita seasoning mix:
(Lawry's Chicken), 1 tsp. 10
(Old El Paso), 1½ tsp. 10
Falafel dishes, mix, dry *(Fantastic Foods)*, ½ cup 250
Farfalle pasta dish mix, w/Alfredo sauce *(Al Dente)*,
   1 cup 230
Farina, whole-grain (see also "Cereal, cooking/hot"):
dry, 1 oz. 105
cooked, 1 cup 116
Fat, see specific listings
Fava bean, see "Broad bean"
Feijoa, raw, w/skin, 1 medium, 2.3 oz. 25
Fennel, bulb, raw:
8.3-oz. bulb 72
sliced, ½ cup 27
Fennel seed, 1 tsp. 7
Fenugreek seed, 1 tsp. 12
Fettuccine:
dry, see "Noodle, egg" and "Pasta"
refrigerated *(Contadina)*, 1¼ cups 240
refrigerated, regular or spinach *(Di Giorno)*, 2.5 oz. 190
refrigerated, spinach *(Contadina)*, 1¼ cups 260
Fettuccine dishes, mix, dry:
Alfredo sauce *(DeBoles)*, 2.4 oz. 270
curly, cheddar-broccoli sauce *(Annie's)*, ⅔ cup 260
tomato-basil sauce *(DeBoles)*, 2 oz. 240

Fettuccine entree, frozen, 1 pkg., except as noted:
Alfredo *(Banquet* Meal), 9.5 oz. 350
Alfredo *(Healthy Choice),* 8 oz. 250
Alfredo *(Lean Cuisine),* 9 oz. 300
Alfredo *(Marie Callender's* Supreme), ½ of 13-oz. pkg. . . 450
Alfredo *(Stouffer's),* 10 oz. 460
Alfredo, w/garlic bread *(Marie Callender's),* 14 oz. 800
w/broccoli and chicken *(Marie Callender's),* ½ of 13-oz.
    pkg. 410
chicken, see "Chicken entree, frozen"
primavera *(Lean Cuisine),* 10 oz. 270
primavera *(Stouffer's),* 10 oz. 370
primavera, w/tortellini *(Marie Callender's),* ½ of 14-oz.
    pkg. 430
Fig:
fresh, 1 large, 2.3 oz. 47
fresh, 1 medium, 1.8 oz. 37
canned, in syrup, ½ cup 114
dried, 10 figs, 6.6 oz. 477
Filbert:
dried, 1 oz. 179
dry-roasted, 1 oz. 188
oil-roasted, 1 oz. 187
Fillo pastry, frozen *(Apollo),* ⅛ pkg. 180
Fish, see specific listings
"Fish," vegetarian:
frozen *(Worthington),* 2 pieces 180
mix *(Loma Linda* Ocean Platter), ⅓ cup dry 90
Fish entree, frozen (see also specific fish listings):
baked *(Lean Cuisine American Favorites),* 9 oz. 270
w/cheese, salsa *(Oven Poppers),* 4.5-oz. piece 130
fillet, in butter sauce *(Mrs. Paul's),* 1 piece 120
fillet, w/macaroni-cheese *(Stouffer's* Homestyle), 9 oz. . . 430
fillet, baked, 1 piece:
    garlic-herb *(Mrs. Paul's/Van de Kamp's* Crunchy) . . . 150
    lemon pepper *(Mrs. Paul's/Van de Kamp's* Crunchy) . 140
fillet, battered *(Mrs. Paul's),* 1 piece 170
fillet, battered *(Van de Kamp's),* 1 piece 180
fillet, breaded:
    (Mrs. Paul's), 2 pieces 240

(Mrs. Paul's/Van de Kamp's Crisp & Healthy),
2 pieces 150
(Van de Kamp's), 2 pieces 280
cornmeal *(Mrs. Paul's/Van de Kamp's Country),*
1 piece 180
w/fries *(Van de Kamp's Fish 'n Fries),* 6.6 oz. 380
fillet, grilled, 1 piece:
garlic butter or Italian herb *(Mrs. Paul's/Van de*
Kamp's) 130
lemon pepper *(Mrs. Paul's/Van de Kamp's)* 130
herb baked *(Healthy Choice),* 10.9 oz. 340
lemon pepper *(Healthy Choice),* 10.7 oz. 320
nuggets, battered *(Van de Kamp's),* 8 pieces 280
portions, battered *(Mrs. Paul's),* 1 piece 160
portions, battered *(Van de Kamp's),* 1 piece 180
portions, breaded *(Mrs. Paul's),* 2 pieces 190
w/shrimp, crab, vegetables *(Oven Poppers),* 4.5-oz.
piece 200
w/spinach, cheese *(Oven Poppers),* 4.5-oz. piece 160
sticks *(Banquet),* 6.6 oz. 290
sticks, battered *(Mrs. Paul's),* 6 pieces 270
sticks, battered *(Van de Kamp's),* 6 pieces 260
sticks, breaded, 6 pieces, except as noted:
(Mrs. Paul's) 210
(Mrs. Paul's/Van de Kamp's Crisp & Healthy) 180
(Mrs. Paul's Value Pack) 220
(Van de Kamp's) 290
(Van de Kamp's Snack/Value Pack) 260
mini *(Van de Kamp's),* 13 pieces 250
Fish seasoning and coating mix *(Shake'n Bake),*
¼ pkt. 70
Flan, see "Pudding"
Flatfish, meat only:
raw, 4 oz. 104
baked, broiled, or microwaved, 4 oz. 133
Flavor enhancer *(Ac'cent),* ⅛ tsp. 0
Flax powder *(Arrowhead Mills Nutri Flax),* 2 tbsp. 70
Flax seeds *(Arrowhead Mills),* 3 tbsp. 140
Flounder:
fresh, see "Flatfish"

frozen *(Van de Kamp's)*, 4-oz. fillet 110
Flounder entree, frozen:
au gratin *(Oven Poppers)*, 5-oz. piece 220
breaded, fillet *(Mrs. Paul's)*, 2.8-oz. piece 170
breaded fillet *(Van de Kamp's)*, 4-oz. piece 230
stuffed w/broccoli and cheese *(Oven Poppers)*, 5 oz. . . . 150
stuffed w/crab *(Oven Poppers)*, 5 oz. 250
stuffed w/garlic, shrimp, almonds *(Oven Poppers)*, 5 oz. . 250
Flour, see "Wheat flour" and specific listings
Frankfurter, 1 link, except as noted:
(Boar's Head Natural Casing/Skinless) 150
(Healthy Choice Low Fat), 1.4 oz. 60
(Healthy Choice Low Fat/Bunsize), 1.8 oz. 70
(Oscar Mayer Little Wieners), 6 links 180
(Oscar Mayer Wieners) 150
(Oscar Mayer Big & Juicy Original Wieners) 240
(Oscar Mayer Bun-Length Wieners) 190
(Oscar Mayer Free Hot Dogs) 40
(Oscar Mayer Light Wieners) 110
beef *(Boar's Head* Lite) 90
beef *(Boar's Head* Natural Casing) 160
beef *(Boar's Head* Skinless) 120
beef *(Healthy Choice)* 80
beef *(Oscar Mayer)* 140
beef *(Oscar Mayer Big & Juicy* Original) 240
beef *(Oscar Mayer Bun-Length)* 180
beef *(Oscar Mayer Light)* 110
cheese *(Oscar Mayer* Hot Dogs) 140
hot and spicy *(Oscar Mayer* Little Wieners), 6 links 170
hot and spicy *(Oscar Mayer Big & Juicy* Wieners) 220
regular or beef *(Ball Park Franks)* 180
regular or beef *(Ball Park Franks* Fat Free) 45
regular or beef *(Ball Park Lite Franks)* 100
smoked *(Oscar Mayer Big & Juicy* Smokie) 220
turkey *(Ball Park Franks* Fat Free) 40
"Frankfurter," vegetarian, 1 link, except as noted:
canned *(Loma Linda* Big) 110
canned *(Loma Linda* Linketts) 70
canned *(Worthington Super Links)* 110
canned *(Worthington Veja Links)* 50

frozen *(Morningstar Farms Original)* 80
frozen *(Natural Touch Vege Frank)* 100
frozen *(Worthington Leanies)* 100
frozen, corn *(Loma Linda/Morningstar Farms)* 150
Frankfurter sandwich, frozen:
(Ball Park Fun Franks), 1 frank, 4 oz. 350
corn dog *(Ball Park)*, 1 piece 220
corn dog, beef *(Ball Park)*, 1 piece 220
beef *(Ball Park Fun Franks)*, 1 frank, 4 oz. 340
French toast, frozen *(Aunt Jemima)*, 2 pieces 240
Frog's legs, meat only, raw, 4 oz. 83
Frosting, ready-to-spread, 2 tbsp.:
banana creme or caramel pecan *(Pillsbury Creamy*
  Supreme) 150
butter cream *(Creamy Deluxe)* 150
caramel pecan *(Pillsbury Creamy Supreme)* 150
cherry *(Creamy Deluxe)* 140
chocolate:
  (Creamy Deluxe) 130
  (Pillsbury Creamy Supreme) 140
  (Sweet Rewards) 120
  (Whipped Deluxe) 100
  dark *(Creamy Deluxe)* 140
  dark *(Pillsbury Creamy Supreme)* 130
  milk *(Creamy Deluxe)* 150
  milk *(Sweet Rewards)* 120
  milk *(Whipped Deluxe)* 100
  milk, swirl, w/fudge glaze *(Pillsbury Creamy*
    Supreme) 140
  milk or mocha *(Pillsbury Creamy Supreme)* 140
  w/stars *(Creamy Deluxe)* 140
coconut pecan *(Creamy Deluxe)* 140
coconut pecan *(Pillsbury Creamy Supreme)* 160
cream cheese *(Creamy Deluxe)* 140
cream cheese *(Pillsbury Creamy Supreme)* 150
cream cheese *(Whipped Deluxe)* 100
creamy candy *(Pillsbury Creamy Supreme)* 150
fudge, hot *(Pillsbury Creamy Supreme)* 140
Funfetti, chocolate *(Pillsbury Creamy Supreme)* 140
lemon *(Creamy Deluxe)* 140

Frosting *(cont.)*
lemon *(Whipped Deluxe)* 100
lemon cream *(Pillsbury Creamy Supreme)* 150
rainbow chip *(Creamy Deluxe)* 140
sour cream, chocolate or white *(Creamy Deluxe)* 150
strawberry cream cheese *(Creamy Deluxe)* 150
strawberry creme *(Pillsbury Creamy Supreme)* 150
vanilla *(Creamy Deluxe)* 140
vanilla *(Pillsbury Creamy Supreme)* 150
vanilla *(Whipped Deluxe)* 100
vanilla, French *(Pillsbury Creamy Supreme)* 160
vanilla swirl, w/fudge glaze *(Pillsbury Creamy Supreme)* . 150
white, fluffy *(Whipped Deluxe)* 100
white chocolate *(Creamy Deluxe)* 140
Fructose *(Estee)*, 1 tsp. 16
Fruit, see specific listings
Fruit, mixed, canned (see also "Fruit cocktail"):
(Del Monte Very Cherry), ½ cup 90
in juice *(Del Monte* Fruit Naturals Chunky), ½ cup 60
in juice *(Del Monte* Fruit Naturals Cup), 4 oz. 50
in extra light syrup *(Del Monte* Lite Chunky), ½ cup 60
in extra light syrup *(Del Monte* Lite Cup), 4 oz. 50
in light syrup, California *(Del Monte* Orchard Select),
 ½ cup 80
in light syrup, tropical *(Del Monte)*, ½ cup 80
in heavy syrup *(Del Monte* Chunky), ½ cup 100
in heavy syrup *(Del Monte* Cup), 4 oz. 80
Fruit bar, frozen (see also "Yogurt bar"), 1 bar:
(Starburst Single) 80
all flavors *(Mr. Freeze)* 50
all flavors *(Mr. Freeze* Sugar Free) 20
coconut *(Edy's/Dreyer's)* 130
lemon and strawberry *(Real Fruit)* 80
lemon lemonade *(Minute Maid)* 90
lime, raspberry kiwi, or strawberry *(Edy's/Dreyer's)* 80
Fruit cocktail, canned, ½ cup:
in juice *(Del Monte* Fruit Naturals) 60
in extra light syrup *(Del Monte* Lite) 60
in heavy syrup *(Del Monte)* 100
Fruit dip, see "Apple dip" and "Chocolate dip"

Fruit drink blends (see also "Soft drinks" and specific listings):

(Capri Sun Mountain Cooler), 6.75 fl. oz.	100
(Capri Sun Pacific Cooler), 6.75 fl. oz.	110
(Capri Sun Surfer Cooler), 6.75 fl. oz.	100
(Dole Fruit Fiesta), 8 fl. oz.	140
(Dole Tropical Breeze), 8 fl. oz.	120
(Fruitopia Fruit Integration), 8 fl. oz.	111
(Fruitopia Tropical Temptation), 8 fl. oz.	107
(Season's Best Medley), 8 fl. oz.	130
berry or cherry *(Capri Sun)*, 6.75 fl. oz.	100
grape *(Capri Sun)*, 6.75 fl. oz.	110
orange or punch *(Capri Sun)*, 6.75 fl. oz.	100
punch *(Capri Sun Maui Punch)*, 6.75 fl. oz.	110
punch *(Capri Sun Safari Punch)*, 6.75 fl. oz.	100
punch *(Dole)*, 10 fl. oz.	160
punch *(Tropicana)*, 8 fl. oz.	130
punch or tropical *(Tropicana Twister)*, 8 fl. oz.	140
strawberry *(Capri Sun Strawberry Cooler)*, 6.75 fl. oz.	100
tropical *(V8 Splash)*, 8 fl. oz.	110

Fruit drink, mix*, 8 fl. oz.:

punch *(Kool-Aid* Tropical)	100
punch *(Kool-Aid* Tropical Presweetened)	60

Fruit juice blends (see also specific listings), 8 fl. oz.:

(Dole)	160
(Minute Maid)	119
apple, blueberry, strawberry *(Hood* 50% Juice)	120
apple, cranberry, raspberry *(Hood* 30% Juice)	130
apple, cranberry, raspberry *(Minute Maid)*	123
punch *(Hood)*	130
punch *(Minute Maid)*	112
punch *(Ocean Spray)*	130
punch, Concord *(Minute Maid)*	127

Fruit pectin *(Sure•Jell)*, 1/4 tsp. 5
Fruit protector *(Ever-Fresh)*, 1/4 tsp. 5

Fruit snack (see also specific fruit listings), all varieties:

(Fruit By the Foot), 3/4-oz. roll	80
(Fruit Gushers), .9-oz. pouch	90
(Fruit Roll-Ups), 1/2-oz. roll	50
(Fruit String Thing), 3/4-oz. pouch	80

Fruit spreads (see also "Jam and preserves"), 1 tbsp.:

all flavors *(Kraft)* 50

all flavors *(Kraft* Reduced Calorie) 20

Fruit syrup, see specific listings

Fruit-nut mix, see "Trail mix"

Fudge, see "Candy"

Fudge topping, see "Chocolate topping"

Fusilli dishes mix, dry, w/garlic herb sauce

(Al Dente), ¾ cup 230

G

FOOD AND MEASURE

CALORIES

Gai choy, see "Cabbage, mustard"
Garbanzo beans, ½ cup, except as noted:
dried *(Arrowhead Mills)*, ¼ cup 170
dried, boiled 134
canned *(Allens/East Texas Fair)* 120
canned *(Green Giant/Joan of Arc)* 110
canned *(Old El Paso)* 100
canned *(Progresso)* 110
canned *(Progresso* Chickpeas) 120
canned *(Seneca)* 110
Garbanzo flour *(Arrowhead Mills)*, ¼ cup 90
Garlic:
(Frieda's Elephant), 1 tbsp. 5
1 clove, .1 oz. 4
chopped in oil or crushed *(Christopher Ranch)*, 1 tsp. . . . 10
pickled *(Christopher Ranch)*, 3 pieces 5
roasted *(Christopher Ranch)*, 2–3 cloves 10
Garlic basting sauce *(Tabasco)*, 1 tbsp. 20
Garlic pepper, 1 tsp. 8
Garlic powder or salt *(Lawry's)*, ¼ tsp. 0
Garlic spread:
(Lawry's Concentrate), 2 tsp. 50
(Lawry's Ready-to-Spread), 1 tbsp. 100
and herb *(McCormick)*, ½ tbsp. 45
Gefilte fish, drained, 1 piece:
in jelled broth *(Manischewitz)* 80
sweet *(Manischewitz)* 90
whitefish and pike *(Manischewitz)* 50
Gelatin dessert, ½ cup:
all flavors, except strawberry *(Kraft Handi-Snacks)* 80
all flavors *(Jell-O)* 80
all flavors *(Jell-O* Sugar Free) 10
strawberry *(Kraft Handi-Snacks)* 80

Gelatin dessert mix*:
all flavors *(Jell-O)*, ½ cup 80
all flavors *(Jell-O* Sugar Free), ½ cup 10
strawberry *(D-Zerta)*, ½ cup 10
strawberry *(Jell-O 1-2-3)*, ⅔ cup 130
Gelatin drink mix, orange *(Knox)*, 1 pkt. 40
Gil choy *(Frieda's)*, 1 tbsp. 0
Ginger, trimmed root:
(Frieda's), 1 tbsp. 0
sliced, ¼ cup 17
sliced *(Ka•Me)*, 20 pieces, .5 oz. 0
Ginger, candied or crystallized:
(Christopher Ranch), 1 tsp. 15
(Frieda's), 9 pieces, 1 oz. 100
Ginger, ground, 1 tsp. 6
Ginger, pickled, Japanese, 1 oz. 10
Ginkgo nut, shelled:
canned, drained, 1 oz. 32
dried, 1 oz. 99
Glaze, pie, strawberry *(Smucker's)*, 2 oz. 80
Glaze, ham, see "Ham glaze"
Glaze mix, see "Seasoning and coating mix"
Gluten, see "Wheat flour"
Goat, meat only, roasted, 4 oz. 162
Godfather's Pizza, 1 slice:
original crust:
cheese, mini, ¼ pie 131
cheese, medium, ⅛ pie 231
cheese, large, ¹⁄₁₀ pie 258
cheese, jumbo, ¹⁄₁₀ pie 382
combo, mini, ¼ pie 176
combo, medium, ⅛ pie 306
combo, large, ¹⁄₁₀ pie 338
combo, jumbo, ¹⁄₁₀ pie 503
golden crust:
cheese, medium, ⅛ pie 212
cheese, large, ¹⁄₁₀ pie 242
combo, medium, ⅛ pie 271
combo, large, ¹⁄₁₀ pie 305

Goose, roasted:

meat w/skin, 4 oz. 346

meat only, 4 oz. 270

Goose fat, 1 oz. 255

Goose liver, see "Liver" and "Pâté"

Gooseberries, fresh, 1/2 cup:

Grain, see specific listings

Grain dishes, mix, 4, w/wild rice *(Fantastic Foods
    Healthy Complements),* 1/2 cup 160

Granadilla, see "Passion fruit"

Granola, see "Cereal"

Granola and cereal bar (see also "Snack bar"), 1 bar:

all fruit varieties *(Health Valley Healthy Breakfast Bakes)* . 110

all fruit varieties *(Kellogg's Nutri-Grain)* 140

all varieties *(Entenmann's)* 140

apple *(Health Valley Apple Bakes)* 70

apple or apricot *(Health Valley* Fruit Bar) 140

blueberry filled, oat bran flakes w/*(Health Valley* Cereal
    Bar) 110

brownie, fudge-filled *(Health Valley)* 110

cheesecake, all varieties *(Health Valley)* 160

chocolate, creme filled, all varieties *(Health Valley*
    Sandwich Bar) 150

chocolate or chocolate chip *(Kudos)* 120

chocolate chip *(Health Valley* Granola Bar) 140

chocolate chip squares *(Kellogg's Rice Krispies Treats)* . . 90

date *(Health Valley* Fruit Bar) 140

date *(Health Valley Date Bakes)* 70

granola, all fruit varieties *(Health Valley)* 140

(Kellogg's Rice Krispies Treats) 90

marshmallow, all varieties *(Health Valley)* 90

oat bran, raisin cinnamon *(Health Valley* Fruit Bar) 160

peanut butter *(Kudos)* 130

raisin *(Health Valley* Fruit Bar) 140

raisin *(Health Valley Raisin Bakes)* 70

raisin apple filled, raisin bran flakes w/ *(Health Valley*
    Cereal Bar) 110

raspberry, red *(Health Valley Healthy Breakfast Bakes)* . . . 110

rice, crispy, all fruit varieties *(Health Valley)* 110

Granola and cereal bar *(cont.)*
strawberry filled, fiber 7 flakes w/ *(Health Valley* Cereal
Bar) 110
Grape, fresh, ½ cup, except as noted:
American type (slipskin), 10 medium 15
American type (slipskin), peeled and seeded 29
champagne *(Frieda's),* 5 oz. 100
European type (adherent skin), seedless, 10 medium 36
European type (adherent skin), seedless or seeded 57
Grape, canned, seedless, in heavy syrup, ½ cup 94
Grape drink blend:
(Fruitopia the Grape Beyond), 8 fl. oz. 119
(Tropicana), 11.5 fl. oz. 200
berry *(Tropicana Twister),* 8 fl. oz. 130
Grape drink mix, 8 fl. oz.*:
(Kool-Aid) 100
(Kool-Aid Presweetened) 60
(Kool-Aid Sugar Free) 5
Grape juice *(Season's Best),* 8 fl. oz. 160
Grape leaves, in jars, *(Krinos),* 1 leaf 5
Grapefruit, fresh:
(Ocean Spray), 2 oz. 50
pink or red, California/Arizona, ½ medium, 3¾″ 46
pink or red, California/Arizona, sections w/juice, ½ cup . . 43
pink or red, Florida, ½ medium, 3¾″ 37
pink or red, Florida, sections w/juice, ½ cup 34
white, California, ½ medium, 3¾″ 43
white, California, sections w/juice, ½ cup 42
white, Florida, ½ medium, 3¾″, or ½ cup sections w/
juice 38
Grapefruit, canned, or chilled, in juice, ½ cup 46
Grapefruit drink, 8 fl. oz.:
pink *(Tropicana Twister)* 120
pink *(Tropicana Twister* Light) 40
ruby red *(Ocean Spray)* 130
ruby red *(Season's Best)* 130
ruby red *(Tropicana Twister)* 130
Grapefruit drink blend, ruby red, 8 fl. oz.:
mango or tangerine *(Ocean Spray)* 130
tangerine *(Tropicana Twister)* 130

Grapefruit drink mix*, pink *(Crystal Light)*, 8 fl. oz. 5
Grapefruit juice, 8 fl. oz., except as noted:
fresh, 6 fl. oz. 72
golden *(Tropicana Pure Premium)* 90
pink *(Minute Maid)* 124
pink *(Ocean Spray)* 110
ruby red *(Season's Best)* 90
ruby red *(Tropicana Pure Premium)* 100
white *(Ocean Spray)* 100
Grapefruit juice blend, orange *(Tropicana Pure
    Premium)*, 8 fl. oz. 110
Gravy, see specific listings
Gravy seasoning (see also "Browning sauce")
(Kitchen Bouquet), 1 tsp. 15
Great northern bean, 1/2 cup:
dried, boiled 104
canned *(Allens)* 100
canned *(Green Giant/Joan of Arc)* 100
canned *(Seneca)* 150
canned, w/sausage *(Trappey's)* 100
Green bean, fresh:
raw, 1/2 cup 17
boiled, drained, 1/2 cup 22
Green bean, canned, 1/2 cup:
(Allens Shell Outs) 30
(Green Giant Kitchen Sliced) 20
all styles *(Seneca/Seneca* No Salt) 25
all styles, except seasoned *(Del Monte)* 20
whole *(Green Giant)* 25
cut *(Allens* No Salt) 15
cut *(Allens/Sunshine/GaBelle/Alma/Crest Top)* 30
cut *(Green Giant/Green Giant* 50% Less Sodium) 20
French style *(Allens)* 25
French style *(Green Giant)* 20
Italian cut *(Allens)* 35
Italian cut *(Del Monte)* 30
w/potatoes *(Allens/Sunshine)* 35
seasoned, french style *(Del Monte)* 20
Green bean, frozen:
(Seneca), 3/4 cup 30

Green bean, frozen *(cont.)*

whole *(Seabrook)*, ³/₄ cup 25

cut *(Cascadian Farm)*, ²/₃ cup 40

cut *(Green Giant)*, ³/₄ cup 25

cut *(Green Giant Harvest Fresh)*, ²/₃ cup 25

w/Szechuan sauce *(Cascadian Farm)*, 1 cup 60

Green bean combinations, frozen:

(Green Giant Casserole), ²/₃ cup 130

w/almonds *(Cascadian Farm)*, ²/₃ cup 70

w/almonds *(Green Giant)*, ²/₃ cup 60

mushroom casserole *(Stouffer's* 36 oz.), ¹/₂ cup 130

mushroom w/garlic sauce *(Cascadian Farm)*, ³/₄ cup 90

Green peas, see "Peas, green"

Greens, mixed, canned *(Allens/Sunshine)*, ¹/₂ cup 30

Grenadine syrup *(Trader Vic's)*, 1 fl. oz. 90

Grilling sauce, chili pepper spice or sweet 'n smoky

(Old El Paso), 2 tbsp. 60

Grits, see "Corn grits"

Grog mixer *(Trader Vic's* Navy), 2 oz. 124

Ground cherry, ¹/₂ cup 37

Grouper, meat only:

raw, 4 oz. 104

baked, broiled, or microwaved, 4 oz. 134

Guacamole (see also "Avocado dip") *(Calavo)*, 2 tbsp. . . 60

Guava:

1 medium, 4 oz. 45

strawberry, ¹/₂ cup 85

Guava drink *(Mauna La'i* Island), 8 fl. oz. 130

Guava sauce, cooked, ¹/₂ cup 43

Guinea hen, raw:

meat w/skin, 4 oz. 179

meat only, 4 oz. 125

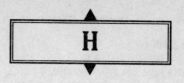

H

FOOD AND MEASURE   **CALORIES**

Haddock, meat only:
raw, 4 oz. 99
baked, broiled, or microwaved, 4 oz. 127
smoked, 4 oz. 132
Haddock entree, fillet, frozen:
battered *(Van de Kamp's),* 2 pieces 260
breaded *(Mrs. Paul's* Premium), 1 piece 230
breaded *(Van de Kamp's),* 2 pieces 280
breaded *(Van de Kamp's* Premium), 1 piece 220
Hake, see "Whiting"
Halibut, meat only, 4 oz.:
Atlantic and Pacific, raw 124
Atlantic and Pacific, baked, broiled, or microwaved 159
Greenland, raw, 4 oz. 211
Greenland, baked, broiled, or microwaved 271
Halibut entree, frozen, fillet, battered *(Van de Kamp's),*
   3 pieces 300
Halvah, chocolate *(Joyva),* 1.75 oz. 340
Ham, fresh, roasted, meat only:
whole leg, lean w/fat, 4 oz. 333
whole leg, lean w/fat, chopped or diced, 1 cup 411
whole leg, lean only, 4 oz. 249
whole leg, lean only, chopped or diced, 1 cup 309
rump half, lean w/fat, 4 oz. 311
rump half, lean only, 4 oz. 251
shank half, lean w/fat, 4 oz. 344
shank half, lean only, 4 oz. 244
Ham, cured:
whole leg, lean w/fat, unheated, 4 oz. 279
whole leg, roasted, 4 oz. 276
whole leg, roasted, chopped or diced, 1 cup 341
whole leg, lean only, unheated, 4 oz. 167
whole leg, lean only, roasted, 4 oz. 178
boneless (11% fat), unheated, 4 oz. 206

Ham, cured *(cont.)*
boneless (11% fat), roasted, 4 oz. 202
boneless, extra lean (5% fat), unheated, 4 oz. 149
boneless, extra lean (5% fat), roasted, 4 oz. 164
Ham, refrigerated:
slice *(Boar's Head Sweet Slice)*, 3 oz. 110
slice *(Oscar Mayer)*, 3 oz. 80
steak *(Oscar Mayer)*, 2 oz. 60
"Ham," vegetarian, frozen *(Worthington Wham)*,
  2 slices 80
Ham entree, frozen, 1 pkg.:
and cheese *(Healthy Choice Hearty Handfuls)*, 6.1 oz. . . . 320
steak, honey-smoked, w/macaroni and cheese *(Marie
  Callender's)*, 14 oz. 490
Ham glaze:
(Boar's Head), 2 tbsp. 120
(Crosse & Blackwell), 1 tbsp. 30
Ham lunch meat, 2 oz., except as noted:
(Black Bear Lower Sodium) 50
(Boar's Head Deluxe) 60
(Boar's Head Deluxe Lower Sodium) 50
(Deli Delight) 60
(Healthy Choice Variety Pack), 1-oz. slice 30
(Healthy Deli Deluxe) 60
(Healthy Deli Tavern) 60
(Oscar Mayer Lower Sodium), 3 slices, 2.2 oz. 70
baked *(Healthy Choice)*, 1-oz. slice 30
baked *(Healthy Choice Deli-Thin)*, 6 slices, 1.9 oz. 60
baked *(Oscar Mayer)*, 3 slices, 2.2 oz. 70
baked *(Oscar Mayer Free)*, 3 slices, 1.7 oz. 35
Black Forest *(Healthy Deli)* 60
boiled *(Oscar Mayer)*, 3 slices, 2.2 oz. 60
cappicola *(Boar's Head Cappy)* 60
cappicola *(Healthy Deli Cappi)* 60
cinnamon apple *(Healthy Deli)* 70
chopped *(Oscar Mayer)*, 1-oz. slice 50
cooked *(Alpine Lace)* 60
cooked *(Healthy Choice)* 60
fresh, seasoned *(Boar's Head)* 80
glazed *(Healthy Deli)* 60

honey *(Alpine Lace)* 60
honey *(Healthy Choice)* 60
honey *(Healthy Deli)* 60
honey *(Oscar Mayer)*, 3 slices, 2.2 oz. 70
honey *(Oscar Mayer Free)*, 3 slices, 1.7 oz. 35
honey, maple *(Healthy Choice)* 60
jalapeño *(Healthy Deli)* 60
loaf *(Diet Delight)* 150
maple *(Healthy Deli Vermont)* 60
maple glazed *(Black Bear)* 60
maple glazed *(Boar's Head)* 60
pepper *(Healthy Deli)* 60
prosciutto, see "Prosciutto"
smoked *(Healthy Choice)* 60
smoked *(Oscar Mayer)*, 3 slices, 2.2 oz. 60
smoked *(Oscar Mayer Free)*, 3 slices, 1.7 oz. 35
smoked, double *(Healthy Deli)*, 2 oz. 60
spiced *(Boar's Head)*, 2 oz. 120
Virginia *(Black Bear)* 50
Virginia *(Boar's Head)* 60
Virginia *(Deli Delight)* 70
Virginia *(Healthy Choice)* 60
Virginia smoked or regular *(Healthy Deli)* 60
Ham spread, ¼ cup:
deviled *(Underwood)* 160
honey *(Underwood)* 140
Ham and cheese loaf *(Oscar Mayer)*, 1-oz. slice 70
Ham and cheese pocket, frozen, 1 piece:
(Big Stuffs), 5.4 oz. 420
(Deli Stuffs), 4.5 oz. 340
(Hot Pockets), 4.5 oz. 320
cheddar *(Croissant Pockets)*, 4.5 oz. 320
cheddar *(Lean Pockets)*, 4.5 oz. 270
melt *(Hot Pockets Toaster Breaks)*, 2.1 oz. 180
Ham and Swiss croissant, frozen *(Sara Lee)*, 1 piece . . . 300
"Hamburger," vegetarian, see "Burger, vegetarian"
Hamburger entree mix, 1 cup*, except as noted:
beef barbecue *(Hamburger Helper)* 320
beef pasta *(Hamburger Helper)* 270
beef Romanoff or beef taco *(Hamburger Helper)* 280

Hamburger entree mix *(cont.)*
beef stew *(Hamburger Helper)* 260
beef teriyaki *(Hamburger Helper)* 290
cheddar and bacon *(Hamburger Helper)* 330
cheddar and broccoli *(Hamburger Helper)* 350
cheddar melt *(Hamburger Helper)* 310
cheddar spirals *(Hamburger Helper* Reduced Sodium) . . . 300
cheese, nacho *(Hamburger Helper)* 320
cheese, three *(Hamburger Helper)* 340
cheeseburger macaroni *(Hamburger Helper)* 360
cheesy hash browns *(Hamburger Helper)* 400
cheesy shells *(Hamburger Helper)* 330
chili macaroni *(Hamburger Helper)* 290
fettuccine Alfredo or zesty Italian *(Hamburger Helper)* . . . 300
Italian herb *(Hamburger Helper* Reduced Sodium) 270
Italian Parmesan w/rigatoni *(Hamburger Helper)* 300
lasagna *(Hamburger Helper)* 270
lasagna, 4-cheese *(Hamburger Helper)* 330
meat loaf *(Hamburger Helper)*, 1/6 loaf* 270
meaty spaghetti and cheese *(Hamburger Helper)* 290
Mexican, zesty *(Hamburger Helper)* 280
mushroom and wild rice *(Hamburger Helper)* 310
Pizzabake (Hamburger Helper), 1/6 pan* 270
pizza pasta or potatoes au grain *(Hamburger Helper)* . . . 280
potato Stroganoff *(Hamburger Helper)* 250
ravioli or rice Oriental *(Hamburger Helper)* 280
ravioli w/cheese topping *(Hamburger Helper)* 310
Salisbury *(Hamburger Helper)* 270
spaghetti *(Hamburger Helper)* 270
Stroganoff *(Hamburger Helper)* 320
Swedish meatballs *(Hamburger Helper)* 290
Southwestern beef *(Hamburger Helper* Reduced
    Sodium) 300
Hard sauce, brandied *(Crosse & Blackwell)*, 2 tbsp. 180
Hazelnut, see "Filbert"
Head cheese:
(Boar's Head), 2 oz. 99
(Oscar Mayer), 1-oz. slice 50
Herbs, see specific listings

Herring, fresh, 4 oz.:
Atlantic, meat only, raw 180
Atlantic, baked, broiled, or microwaved 230
lake, see "Cisco"
Pacific, meat only, raw 224
Pacific, baked, broiled, or microwaved 284
Herring, canned, see "Sardine"
Herring, kippered, Atlantic, 2 oz. 123
Herring, pickled, Atlantic, 2 oz. 149
Herring salad, chopped *(Blue Ridge Farms),* ⅓ cup . . . 150
Hickory nut, dried, shelled, 1 oz. 187
Hoisin sauce *(Ka•Me),* 2 tbsp. 45
Homestyle gravy mix *(Pillsbury),* ¼ cup* 15
Hominy, canned, ½ cup:
golden or Mexican *(Allens/Uncle William)* 120
white *(Allens/Uncle William)* 100
Hominy grits, see "Corn grits"
Honey *(Aunt Sue's/Grandma's/Sue Bee),* 1 tbsp. 60
Honey butter, see "Butter, flavored"
Honey loaf, see "Lunch meat"
Honey mustard, see "Mustard"
Honey mustard sauce:
(Rice Road) 20
Dijon *(World Harbors* Mont St. Michel), 2 tbsp. 30
Honey roll sausage, beef, 1 oz. 52
Honeycomb, strained *(Frieda's),* 1 oz. 86
Honeydew:
¹⁄₁₀ melon, 7″ × 2″ 46
pulp, cubed, ½ cup 30
Horseradish, fresh:
leafy tips, boiled, drained, ½ cup 13
pods, boiled, drained, ½ cup 21
Horseradish, prepared, 1 tsp., except as noted:
(Heluva Good) 0
(Kraft) 0
w/beets *(Gold's)* 0
mustard *(Heluva* Good) 6
Horseradish root *(Frieda's),* 1 tbsp. 0
Horseradish sauce *(Sauceworks),* 1 tsp. 20
Hot buttered rum, batter *(Trader Vic's),* 1 oz. 136

Hot dog, see "Frankfurter"
Hot dog sauce, see "Chili sauce"
Hot fudge sauce, see "Chocolate topping"
Hot sauce, see "Pepper sauce" and specific listings
Hubbard squash:
raw *(Frieda's)*, ¾ cup, 3 oz. 35
baked, cubed, ½ cup 51
boiled, drained, mashed, ½ cup 35
Hummus, 2 tbsp., except as noted:
(Sabra Chumus), 1 oz. 69
chili pepper *(Yorgo)* 50
cucumber dill *(Athenos)* 60
garlic, extra *(Yorgo)* 35
garlic, roasted *(Athenos)* 50
lemon pepper *(Yorgo)* 50
olive, black *(Athenos)* 50
red pepper, roasted *(Athenos)* 60
scallion *(Athenos)* 50
tahini *(Yorgo)* 50
tahini *(Sabra)*, 1 oz. 80
vegetable tahini *(Yorgo)* 45
Hummus dip mix, dry *(Fantastic Foods)*, 2 tbsp. 60
Hush puppy mix *(Martha White)*, ¼ cup fried* 300
Hyacinth bean, ½ cup:
fresh, boiled, drained 22
dried, boiled 114

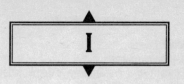

I

FOOD AND MEASURE   **CALORIES**

Ice, lemonade or strawberry *(Minute Maid* Cup),
    12 fl. oz. 300
Ice bar, see "Fruit bar, frozen"
Ice cream, ½ cup:
amaretto *(Häagen-Dazs DiSaronno)* 260
apple crisp *(Edy's* Homemade) 150
apple pie *(Edy's/Dreyer's Grand* Limited Edition) 140
banana cream pie *(Edy's/Dreyer's* Homemade) 130
banana nut or banana split *(Blue Bell)* 170
banana pudding *(Blue Bell)* 190
banana split *(Blue Bell* Diet/Light) 110
banana and chocolate *(Edy's/Dreyer's Grand* Light
    Chiquita) 110
(Ben & Jerry's Cherry Garcia) 260
(Ben & Jerry's Chubby Hubby) 350
(Ben & Jerry's Chunky Monkey) 310
(Ben & Jerry's Phish Food) 300
(Ben & Jerry's Wavy Gravy) 340
Black Forest cake *(Blue Bell)* 170
black walnut *(Blue Bell)* 160
black walnut *(Edy's* Homemade) 160
blackberry *(Ben & Jerry's* Cobbler Low Fat) 180
blueberry cheesecake *(Blue Bell)* 160
blueberry cheesecake *(Edy's/Dreyer's Grand* Limited
    Edition) 130
brownie sundae *(Edy's/Dreyer's* Fat Free No Sugar) 110
butter almond *(Breyers)* 170
butter pecan *(Ben & Jerry's)* 330
butter pecan *(Blue Bell* Buttered) 180
butter pecan *(Blue Bell* Buttered Light) 150
butter pecan *(Breyers)* 180
butter pecan *(Breyers Smucker's* Homemade) 170
butter pecan *(Edy's/Dreyer's Grand*/Homemade) 160
butter pecan *(Edy's/Dreyer's Grand* Light) 120

Ice cream *(cont.)*

butter pecan *(Häagen-Dazs)*	310
caramel and cream *(Breyers Smucker's* Homemade)	160
caramel crunch sundae *(Blue Bell)*	190
caramel praline crunch *(Breyers)*	180
caramel praline crunch *(Breyers* Fat Free)	120
caramel praline crunch *(Edy's/Dreyer's* Fat Free)	110
caramel praline pecan *(Breyers* Light)	180
cherry amaretto cordial *(Blue Bell)*	170
cherry chocolate chip *(Edy's Grand)*	150
cherry chocolate chunk *(Edy's/Dreyer's Grand)*	150
cherry cobbler *(Edy's* Homemade)	150
cherry vanilla *(Blue Bell)*	160
cherry vanilla *(Breyers)*	150
cherry vanilla *(Häagen-Dazs)*	240
chocolate *(Blue Bell* Decadence)	190
chocolate *(Breyers)*	160
chocolate *(Edy's/Dreyer's Grand)*	150
chocolate *(Edy's/Dreyer's Grand* Mumbo Jumbo)	170
chocolate *(Häagen-Dazs)*	270
chocolate *(Newman's Own Chocolate Mud Bath)*	190
chocolate, Dutch *(Blue Bell)*	170
chocolate, French *(Breyers* Light)	150
chocolate, milk *(Blue Bell)*	190
chocolate, triple *(Blue Bell)*	180
chocolate, triple *(Edy's/Dreyer's* No Sugar)	100
chocolate almond fudge *(Edy's/Dreyer's Grand* Light)	120
chocolate almond marshmallow *(Blue Bell)*	190
chocolate brownie crunch *(Edy's/Dreyer's* Fat Free)	110
chocolate chip:	
(Edy's/Dreyer's Grand Chips!/Homemade)	170
chocolate *(Häagen-Dazs)*	300
cookie dough *(Ben & Jerry's)*	300
cookie dough *(Blue Bell)*	190
cookie dough *(Breyers)*	180
mint *(Breyers* Light)	140
mint *(Breyers* No Sugar)	100
mint *(Healthy Choice)*	120
regular or mint *(Blue Bell)*	170
regular or mint *(Breyers)*	170

chocolate chunk, double *(Edy's/Dreyer's Homemade)* . . . 190
chocolate cream pie *(Blue Bell)* 180
chocolate fudge *(Edy's/Dreyer's Fat Free)* 110
chocolate fudge, brownie *(Ben & Jerry's)* 280
chocolate fudge, double *(Breyers Homemade)* 180
chocolate fudge mousse *(Edy's/Dreyer's Grand)* 160
chocolate peanut butter *(Edy's Homemade)* 200
chocolate pecan cheesecake *(Blue Bell)* 200
chocolate rainbow *(Breyers)* 120
chocolate sundae *(Blue Bell)* 170
coconut almond fudge chip *(Ben & Jerry's)* 310
coconut cream pie *(Ben & Jerry's Low Fat)* 160
coffee *(Ben & Jerry's Coffee Coffee Buzz Buzz Buzz)* 290
coffee *(Blue Bell)* 160
coffee *(Edy's/Dreyer's Grand)* 140
coffee *(Häagen-Dazs)* 270
coffee *(Newman's Own Giddy Up Coffee)* 170
coffee fudge *(Edy's/Dreyer's Fat Free)* 110
coffee mocha chip *(Häagen-Dazs)* 290
cookie creme de menthe *(Healthy Choice)* 130
cookie chunk *(Edy's/Dreyer's Fat Free)* 110
cookie dough *(Edy's/Dreyer's Grand)* 170
cookie dough *(Edy's/Dreyer's Grand Light)* 130
cookie jar *(Edy's/Dreyer's Grand Limited Edition)* 170
cookies and cream *(Blue Bell)* 180
cookies and cream *(Blue Bell Light)* 120
cookies and cream *(Breyers)* 170
cookies and cream *(Häagen-Dazs)* 270
cookies and cream, mint *(Breyers Fat Free)* 100
cookies and cream, mint *(Dreyer's Grand Light)* 120
cookies and fudge *(Edy's Homemade)* 160
espresso chip *(Edy's Grand)* 150
espresso chip fudge *(Dreyer's Grand Light)* 120
French Silk (Edy's/Dreyer's Grand Light) 120
fruit rainbow *(Breyers)* 140
fudge, vanilla caramel *(Ben & Jerry's)* 300
fudge brownie, double *(Edy's/Dreyer's No Sugar)* 100
fudge brownie, double *(Edy's/Dreyer's Grand)* 170
fudge brownie hot *(Blue Bell)* 200
fudge cake, turtle *(Healthy Choice)* 130

Ice cream *(cont.)*

fudge chunk *(Ben & Jerry's New York Super)* 320
lemon *(Blue Bell)* 150
macadamia nut brittle *(Häagen-Dazs)* 300
marble fudge *(Edy's/Dreyer's Fat Free)* 110
marble fudge *(Edy's/Dreyer's No Sugar)* 90
mint chip *(Häagen-Dazs)* 290
mint chip *(Newman's Own Lovable Mint Chip)* 230
mint chocolate chip, see "chocolate chip," above
mint chocolate cookie *(Ben & Jerry's)* 280
mint fudge *(Dreyer's Fat Free)* 110
mint patty, vanilla/chocolate *(Ben & Jerry's Low Fat)* . . . 170
mocha fudge almond *(Dreyer's Grand)* 170
mocha fudge almond *(Dreyer's Grand Light)* 120
Neapolitan *(Blue Bell)* 160
peach *(Breyers)* 130
peach vanilla *(Blue Bell Homemade)* 180
peach vanilla *(Blue Bell Homemade Light)* 140
peanut butter cup *(Ben & Jerry's)* 380
peanut butter cup *(Blue Bell)* 230
pecan praline *(Newman's Own Pistol Packin' Praline
　　Pecan)* 200
pecan praline and cream *(Blue Bell)* 200
peppermint *(Blue Bell)* 160
peppermint *(Edy's/Dreyer's Grand Limited Edition)* 150
pistachio almond *(Blue Bell)* 170
rocky road *(Blue Bell)* 180
rocky road *(Blue Bell Light)* 110
rocky road *(Breyers)* 180
rocky road *(Edy's/Dreyer's Grand)* 170
rocky road *(Edy's/Dreyer's Grand Light)* 120
rum raisin *(Häagen-Dazs)* 270
S'mores *(Blue Bell)* 180
strawberries and cream *(Breyers Smucker's Homemade)* . 150
strawberries and cream *(Edy's/Dreyer's Homemade)* . . . 130
strawberry *(Blue Bell)* 150
strawberry *(Breyers)* 130
strawberry *(Häagen-Dazs)* 250
strawberry, real *(Edy's/Dreyer's Grand)* 130
strawberry and vanilla *(Blue Bell Homemade)* 160

strawberry and vanilla *(Blue Bell* Homemade Light) 140
strawberry cheesecake *(Blue Bell)* 170
tin roof *(Blue Bell)* 200
toffee crunch *(Ben & Jerry's Heath)* 310
vanilla *(Ben & Jerry's World's Best)* 250
vanilla *(Blue Bell* Country) 160
vanilla *(Blue Bell* French) 170
vanilla *(Blue Bell* Homemade) 180
vanilla *(Blue Bell* Homemade Light) 140
vanilla *(Breyers)* 150
vanilla *(Breyers* Fat Free/No Sugar) 90
vanilla *(Breyers* Light) 120
vanilla *(Dreyer's Grand)* 150
vanilla *(Edy's/Dreyer's* Fat Free) 100
vanilla *(Edy's/Dreyer's* Homemade/*Edy's Grand)* 140
vanilla *(Häagen-Dazs)* 270
vanilla *(Newman's Own Obscene Vanilla Bean)* 170
vanilla, French *(Breyers)* 160
vanilla, French *(Edy's/Dreyer's Grand)* 160
vanilla bean *(Blue Bell)* 190
vanilla bean *(Blue Bell* Diet) 100
vanilla bean *(Edy's Dreyer's Grand)* 140
vanilla chocolate *(Breyers* Take Two) 160
vanilla chocolate *(Edy's Grand)* 150
vanilla chocolate chip *(Häagen-Dazs)* 310
vanilla chocolate strawberry *(Breyers)* 150
vanilla chocolate strawberry *(Breyers* Fat Free) 90
vanilla chocolate strawberry *(Breyers* Light) 120
vanilla fudge *(Häagen-Dazs)* 290
vanilla fudge twirl *(Breyers)* 160
vanilla fudge twirl *(Breyers* Fat Free/No Sugar) 100
vanilla orange sherbet *(Breyers* Take Two) 130
vanilla strawberry *(Breyers* Fat Free Take Two) 80
vanilla Swiss almond *(Häagen-Dazs)* 310
white chocolate almond *(Blue Bell)* 190
"Ice cream," nondairy, 1/2 cup:
cappuccino or carob *(Rice Dream)* 150
cappuccino almond fudge *(Rice Dream* Supreme) 170
carob almond *(Rice Dream)* 170
cherry vanilla *(Rice Dream)* 150

"Ice cream," nondairy *(cont.)*

chocolate or vanilla *(Rice Dream)* 150
chocolate almond or cherry chunk *(Rice Dream*
   Supreme) 170
chocolate chip *(Rice Dream)* 170
chocolate fudge brownie *(Rice Dream* Supreme) 170
cocoa marble fudge *(Rice Dream)* 150
cookie n' dream *(Rice Dream)* 170
espresso bean, double *(Rice Dream* Supreme) 160
mint carob chip *(Rice Dream)* 170
Neapolitan or orange vanilla swirl *(Rice Dream)* 150
peanut butter cup or pralines n' dream *(Rice Dream*
   Supreme) 180
strawberry *(Rice Dream)* 140
vanilla Swiss almond *(Rice Dream)* 180

Ice cream bar, 1 bar:

almond *(Klondike)* 310
(Ben & Jerry's Chunky Monkey) 360
(Ben & Jerry's Phish Stick) 330
(Ben & Jerry's Totally Nuts) 370
cappuccino *(Klondike)* 290
caramel crunch *(Klondike* Multi Pack) 300
chocolate, chocolate or dark *(Klondike* Multi Pack) . . . 290
chocolate w/dark chocolate *(Häagen-Dazs* Multipack) . . . 290
chocolate w/dark chocolate *(Häagen-Dazs* Single) 350
chocolate mousse *(Smart Ones* Lowfat) 40
cookie dough *(Ben & Jerry's)* 420
cookies and cream *(Edy's/Dreyer's)* 250
cookies and cream *(Oreo)* 180
coffee/almond crunch *(Häagen-Dazs* Multipack) 310
coffee/almond crunch *(Häagen-Dazs* Single) 360
(Klondike Krispy Krunch), 5 fl. oz. 300
(Klondike Krunch), 4 fl. oz. 270
(Klondike Original) 290
mint cookie, thin *(Edy's/Dreyer's Girl Scouts)* 280
Neapolitan *(Klondike* Multi Pack) 280
strawberry/white chocolate *(Häagen-Dazs* Multipack) . . . 270
strawberry/white chocolate *(Häagen-Dazs* Single) 320
toffee crunch *(Ben & Jerry's Vanilla Heath)* 330
vanilla *(Ben & Jerry's* Peace Pop) 330

vanilla *(Klondike* Multi Pack) 290
vanilla and almonds *(Edy's/Dreyer's)* 250
vanilla w/almonds *(Häagen-Dazs* Multipack) 320
vanilla w/almonds *(Häagen-Dazs* Single) 370
vanilla w/dark chocolate *(Eskimo Pie)* 160
vanilla w/dark chocolate *(Häagen-Dazs* Multipack) 290
vanilla w/dark chocolate *(Häagen-Dazs* Single) 350
vanilla, w/milk chocolate *(Edy'd/Dreyer's)* 250
vanilla w/milk chocolate *(Eskimo Pie)* 160
vanilla w/milk chocolate *(Häagen-Dazs* Multipack) 280
vanilla w/milk chocolate *(Häagen-Dazs* Single) 330
"Ice cream" bar, nondairy, 1 bar:
carob coated, chocolate/vanilla *(The Rice Dream Bar)* . . . 270
carob coated, strawberry *(The Rice Dream Bar)* 250
chocolate *(Smart Ones* Treat) 100
nut coated, chocolate/vanilla *(The Nutty Rice Dream
    Bar)* 260
Ice cream cake:
(Viennetta Individuals), 1 piece 240
all flavors *(Viennetta),* 2.4-oz. slice 190
Ice cream cone or cup, plain, unfilled, 1 piece:
bowl, waffle *(Keebler)* 50
cone, fudge-dipped *(Keebler)* 35
cone, sugar or waffle *(Keebler)* 50
cup *(Keebler)* 15
Ice cream cone, filled, 1 cone:
caramel *(Klondike)* 310
caramel *(Klondike* Kombo Kones) 320
cookies and cream *(Oreo)* 230
cookies and cream sundae *(Edy's/Dreyer's)* 250
fudge *(Klondike* Kombo Kones) 320
vanilla, w/chocolate and peanuts *(Eskimo Pie)* 210
vanilla fudge sundae *(Edy's/Dreyer's)* 240
"Ice cream" cone, nondairy, chocolate or vanilla
(Rice Dream), 1 cone 270
Ice cream cup, filled, sundae *(Klondike),* 6 fl. oz. 280
Ice cream pie, vanilla w/fudge *(Eskimo Pie Arctic
    Madness),* 1 piece 260
"Ice cream" pie, nondairy, all flavors *(Rice Dream),*
    1 pie 320

Ice cream sandwich, 1 piece:
(*Eskimo Pie*) 160
(*Klondike* Big Bear Fat Free) 130
(*Klondike Choc Burger* Multi Pack) 320
(*Klondike Choc Burger* Single) 350
(*Klondike Choco Taco*) 310
vanilla (*Häagen-Dazs*) 260
vanilla and chocolate (*Häagen-Dazs*) 260
Ice cream and sorbet, see "Sorbet"
Icing, see "Frosting"
Italian cut beans, see "Green beans, canned"
Italian sausage, see "Sausage"
Italian seasoning, 1 tsp. 3

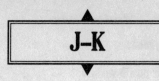

FOOD AND MEASURE   **CALORIES**

Jack-in-the-Box, 1 serving:
breakfast items:
    Breakfast Jack 280
    Country Crock Spread 25
    croissant, sausage 690
    croissant, supreme 520
    grape jelly 40
    hash browns 170
    pancakes, w/bacon 370
    sandwich, sourdough 440
    sandwich, ultimate 620
    syrup 130
burgers:
    cheeseburger, double 460
    cheeseburger, ultimate 1030
    cheeseburger, ultimate, bacon 1150
    hamburger 280
    hamburger w/cheese 320
    Jumbo Jack 590
    Jumbo Jack w/cheese 680
    Sourdough Jack 690
sandwiches:
    chicken 450
    chicken, spicy crispy 560
    chicken Caesar 490
    chicken fajita pita 280
    chicken fillet, grilled 520
    chicken supreme 680
    Philly cheesesteak 520
cheese, American, 1 slice 45
cheese, Swiss style, 1 slice 40
taco 170
taco, monster 270

Jack-in-the-Box (cont.)

finger foods:

bacon cheddar potato wedges	800
chicken breast, 5 pieces	360
chicken (4 pieces) and fries	730
dipping sauce, barbecue or sweet and sour, 1 oz.	45
dipping sauce, buttermilk house, 1 oz.	130
egg rolls, 3 pieces	440
egg rolls, 5 pieces	730
fish and chips	780
jalapeños, stuffed, 7 pieces	530
jalapeños, stuffed, 10 pieces	750
salsa, 1 oz.	10
sour cream, 1.1 oz.	60

salads:

chicken teriyaki bowl	670
garden chicken salad	200
side salad or croutons	50
soy sauce	5

    dressings:

blue cheese	210
buttermilk house	290
Italian, low-cal	25
Thousand Island	250

sides:

fries, regular	350
fries, jumbo	430
fries, super scoop	610
fries, curly, seasoned	410
fries, chili cheese	650
onion rings	460

desserts/shakes:

apple turnover, hot	340
carrot cake	370
cheesecake	320
double fudge cake	300

    shakes, regular:

cappuccino or chocolate	630
Oreo cookie	320
strawberry	640

vanilla 610
Jackfruit, trimmed, 1 oz. 27
Jackfruit, dried *(Frieda's),* ⅓ cup 120
Jalapeño, see "Pepper, jalapeño"
Jalapeño dip (see also "Cheese dip"), 2 tbsp.:
(Kraft) 60
(Old El Paso) 30
Jam and preserves (see also "Fruit spreads"), 1 tbsp.,
  except as noted:
all fruits *(Knott's Berry Farm),* 1 tsp. 18
all fruits *(Smucker's)* 50
grape or red plum *(Kraft)* 60
marmalade, all varieties except orange *(Crosse &*
  Blackwell) 60
marmalade, orange *(Crosse & Blackwell)* 50
strawberry *(Kraft)* 50
Jelly, 1 tbsp.:
all fruits *(Smucker's)* 50
all fruit, except apple and strawberry *(Kraft)* 50
apple or strawberry *(Kraft)* 60
guava or red currant *(Crosse & Blackwell)* 50
mint *(Crosse & Blackwell)* 60
strawberry *(Kraft)* 60
Jerk sauce (see also "Marinade"), 2 tbsp.:
(World Harbors Blue Mountain) 70
dipping *(Helen's Tropical Exotics* Jamaican) 45
Jerk seasoning *(Helen's Tropical Exotics),* 1 tbsp. 30
Jerusalem artichoke:
(Frieda's Sun Choke), ½ cup, 3 oz. 70
sliced, ½ cup 57
Jicama, see "Yam bean tuber"
Jujube, raw, seeded, 1 oz. 22
dried, 1 oz. 81
Jute, boiled, drained, ½ cup 16
Kale, ½ cup, except as noted:
fresh, raw, chopped 17
fresh, boiled, drained, chopped 21
canned *(Allens/Sunshine)* 25
Kale, Chinese *(Frieda's* Gai Lan), 1 cup, 3 oz. 15

Kale, Scotch, ½ cup:
raw, chopped 14
boiled, drained, chopped 18
Kamranga, see "Carambola"
Kamut flakes, see "Cereal"
Kamut flour *(Arrowhead Mills),* ¼ cup 110
Kasha, see "Buckwheat groats"
Ketchup, 1 tbsp., except as noted:
(Heinz) 15
(Muir Glen) 15
(Smucker's) 25
w/horseradish *(Gold's),* 1 tsp. 5
KFC, 1 serving:
chicken, *Original Recipe,* 1 piece:
   breast 400
   drumstick or whole wing 140
   thigh 250
Chicken, *Extra Tasty Crispy,* 1 piece
   breast 470
   drumstick 190
   thigh 370
   whole wing 200
Chicken, *Hot & Spicy,* 1 piece:
   breast 180
   drumstick 190
   thigh 370
   whole wing 210
Chicken, *Tender Roast,* 1 piece:
   breast, w/skin 251
   breast, w/out skin 169
   drumstick, w/skin 97
   drumstick, w/out skin 67
   thigh, w/skin 207
   thigh, w/out skin 106
   wing, w/skin 121
Chicken *Twister* 480
Crispy Strips, Colonel's, 3 pieces 261
Crispy Strips, Spicy Buffalo, 3 pieces 350
Hot Wings, 6 pieces 471
pot pie, chunky chicken 770

sandwich, *Original Recipe* 497
sandwich, BBQ flavored, value 256
sides and vegetables:
    baked beans, BBQ 190
    biscuit, 1 piece 180
    cole slaw, 5 oz. 180
    corn on the cob 150
    cornbread, 1 piece 228
    green beans 45
    macaroni and cheese 180
    Mean Greens 70
    potato salad 230
    potato wedges 280
    potatoes, mashed, w/gravy 120
Kidney beans:
dried *(Arrowhead Mills)*, ¼ cup 160
dried, boiled, ½ cup 112
canned, red, ½ cup:
    (Progresso) 110
    (Seneca) 120
    dark *(Allens/East Texas Fair/Trappy's)* 130
    dark or light *(Brooks)* 120
    dark or light *(Green Giant/Joan of Arc)* 110
    light *(Allens/Trappey's)* 120
    w/bacon, light *(Trappey's New Orleans)* 110
    w/chili gravy or jalapeños *(Trappey's)* 110
white *(Progresso Cannellini)* 100
Kidney beans, sprouted, raw, ½ cup 27
Kidneys, braised, beef, 4 oz. 163
Kielbasa (see also "Polish sausage"), 2 oz.:
(Boar's Head) 120
(Healthy Choice Polska) 70
Kim chee *(Frieda's)*, ¼ cup, 2 oz. 15
Kishka *(Hebrew National)*, 2 oz. 160
Kiwi, fresh, 1 medium, 3.1 oz. 46
Kiwi, dried *(Sonoma)*, 7–8 pieces, 1 oz. 90
Kiwi drink blend, 8 fl. oz.:
(Crazy Kiwi Passion) 130
strawberry *(Chiquita Cocktail)* 120
strawberry *(Ocean Spray)* 120

Knockwurst, 1 link:
(*Ball Park*), 4 oz. 360
beef *(Ball Park)*, 4 oz. 340
beef *(Boar's Head)*, 4 oz. 310
beef *(Shofar)*, 3 oz. 210
Kohlrabi, ½ cup:
raw, sliced, ½ cup 19
boiled, drained, sliced, ½ cup 24
Kumquat:
1 medium, .7 oz. 12
seeded, 1 oz. 18
Kun choy, see "Celery, Chinese"

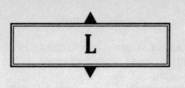

L

FOOD AND MEASURE   **CALORIES**

Lamb, choice, meat only, 4 oz., except as noted:
cubed, leg/shoulder, braised or stewed 253
cubed, leg/shoulder, broiled 211
foreshank, braised, lean w/fat 276
foreshank, braised, lean only 212
ground, raw 320
ground, broiled 321
ground, broiled, 1 cup 328
leg, whole, roasted, lean w/fat 293
leg, whole, lean only 217
leg, shank, roasted, lean w/fat 255
leg, shank, roasted, lean only 204
leg, sirloin, roasted, lean w/fat 331
leg, sirloin, roasted, lean only 231
loin chop, broiled:
    lean w/fat, 2¼ oz. (4.2 oz. raw w/bone) 201
    lean w/fat 358
    lean only, 1.6 oz. (4.2 oz. raw w/bone and fat) 100
    lean only 245
loin, roasted, lean w/fat 350
loin, roasted, lean only 229
rib, broiled, lean w/fat 409
rib, broiled, lean only 266
rib, roasted, lean w/fat 407
rib, roasted, lean only 263
shoulder, whole, braised, lean w/fat 390
shoulder, whole, braised, lean only 321
shoulder, whole, roasted, lean w/fat 313
shoulder, whole, roasted, lean only 231
Lamb, New Zealand, frozen, meat only, 4 oz.:
leg, whole, roasted, lean w/fat 279
leg, whole, roasted, lean only 205
loin chop, broiled, lean w/fat 357
loin chop, broiled, lean only 226

Lamb curry entree, frozen *(Curry Classics),* 10 oz. 480
Lamb's quarters, boiled, drained, chopped, ½ cup 29
Lard, pork, 1 tbsp. 115
Lasagna entree, frozen, 1 pkg., except as noted:
(Amy's), 10.25 oz. 310
(Healthy Choice Roma), 13.5 oz. 400
bake *(Stouffer's),* 10¼ oz. 370
cheese *(Lean Cuisine* Casserole), 10 oz. 270
cheese *(Lean Cuisine* Classic), 11½ oz. 280
cheese, 5 *(Lean Cuisine),* 1/12 of 96-oz. pkg. 210
cheese, 5 *(Stouffer's),* 10¾ oz. 360
cheese, extra *(Marie Callender's),* 1 cup 350
chicken *(Lean Cuisine),* 10 oz. 270
chicken *(Lean Cuisine),* 1/12 of 96-oz. pkg. 230
chicken *(Stouffer's* 39 oz.), 1 cup 320
chicken, cheese, w/chicken scallopini *(Lean Cuisine Cafe
    Classics),* 10 oz. 290
w/Italian sausage *(Marie Callender's),* 15 oz. 710
w/meat sauce *(Banquet),* 9.5 oz. 260
w/meat sauce *(Banquet* Family), 1 cup 100
w/meat sauce *(Lean Cuisine),* 10½ oz. 290
w/meat sauce *(Marie Callender's),* 1 cup 370
w/meat sauce *(Marie Callender's* Family), 1 cup 350
w/meat sauce *(Stouffer's),* 10½ oz. 370
w/meat sauce *(Stouffer's* 21 oz.), 1 cup or ⅓ pkg. 250
w/meat sauce *(Stouffer's* 40 oz.), 1 cup or ⅕ pkg. 270
w/meat sauce *(Stouffer's* 96 oz.), 1 cup or 1/12 pkg. 300
vegetable *(Amy's),* 9.5 oz. 300
vegetable *(Amy's* Family Size), 7 oz. 200
vegetable *(Lean Cuisine),* 10½ oz. 260
vegetable *(Stouffer's),* 10½ oz. 440
vegetable *(Stouffer's* 96 oz.), 1 cup or 1/12 pkg. 330
vegetable, tofu *(Amy's),* 9.5 oz. 300
zucchini *(Healthy Choice),* 13.5 oz. 330
Leek:
fresh *(Frieda's),* 1 cup, 3 oz. 50
fresh, raw, 9.9-oz. leek 76
fresh, boiled, drained, chopped, ½ cup 16
freeze-dried, 1 tbsp. 1
Lemon, fresh, 2⅛" lemon, 3.9 oz. 22

Lemon curd *(Crosse & Blackwell)*, 1 tbsp. 50
Lemon juice, fresh, 1 tbsp. 4
Lemon pepper *(Lawry's)*, ¼ tsp. 0
Lemon sauce, Oriental *(Ka•Me)*, 1 tbsp. 45
Lemonade, 8 fl. oz.:
(Hood). 110
(Sunkist) 120
(Tropicana) 140
(Tropicana Twister Light) 35
(Welch's) 110
pink *(Tropicana Twister)* 120
Lemonade fruit blends *(Fruitopia* Berry Lemonade),
    8 fl. oz. 106
Lemonade, mix*, 8 fl. oz., except as noted:
(Country Time) 70
(Country Time Low Calorie) 5
(Crystal Light) 5
(Kool-Aid) 100
(Kool-Aid Presweetened) 70
(Kool-Aid Sugar Free) 5
punch *(Country Time)* 70
Lemon-lime drink mix*:
(Crystal Light), 8 fl. oz. 5
(Kool-Aid), 8 fl. oz. 100
Lentil:
dry, green or red *(Arrowhead Mills)*, ¼ cup 150
cooked, ½ cup 115
Lentil, sprouted, raw, ½ cup 40
Lentil dishes, canned *(Patak's* Moong Dhal), ½ cup . . . 160
Lentil entree, packaged, w/rice, 1 pkg.:
creamy yellow, w/vegetables *(Tamarind Tree* Channa Dal
    Masala) 340
spicy *(Tamarind Tree* Dal Makhani) 330
Lettuce (see also "Salad blend mix"):
bibb or Boston, 1 head, 5″ diam. 21
bibb or Boston, 2 inner leaves 2
butter *(Dole)*, 1 head 21
cos or romaine, shredded, ½ cup 4
cos or romaine shredded *(Dole)*, 1½ cups 18
iceberg, 1 head, 6″ diam. 70

Lettuce *(cont.)*
iceberg, 1 leaf, .7 oz. 3
iceberg, precut *(Dole),* 3 oz. 15
leaf, shredded *(Dole),* 1½ cups 12
looseleaf, shredded, ½ cup 5
Lima beans, ½ cup, except as noted:
fresh, raw, trimmed 88
fresh, boiled, drained 104
mature, dried *(Frieda's),* ⅓ cup, 3 oz. 120
mature, dried, baby, boiled 115
mature, dried, large, boiled 108
Lima beans, canned, ½ cup, except as noted:
(Green Giant/Joan of Arc Butterbeans) 90
(Seneca) 70
baby *(Allens* Butterbeans) 120
green *(Allens/East Texas Fair* Limas) 120
green *(Del Monte)* 80
green *(Sunshine* Butterbeans) 120
green and white *(Allens* Limas) 110
large *(Allens* Butterbeans) 120
w/bacon, baby green *(Trappey's* Limas) 120
w/bacon, baby white *(Trappey's* Limas) 130
w/sausage, large white *(Trappey's* Butterbeans) 110
Lima beans, frozen:
(Seneca), ⅔ cup 120
baby *(Green Giant Harvest Fresh),* ½ cup 80
baby *(Seabrook),* ½ cup 110
baby, in butter sauce *(Green Giant),* ⅔ cup 120
Fordhook *(Seneca),* ⅔ cup 90
Lime, fresh, 2″-diam. lime 20
peeled, seeded, 1 oz. 9
Lime curd *(Crosse & Blackwell),* 1 tbsp. 50
Lime juice:
fresh, 1 tbsp. 4
sweetened *(Rose's),* 1 tsp. 10
Ling, meat only:
raw, 4 oz. 99
baked, broiled, or microwaved, 4 oz. 126
Ling cod, meat only:
raw, 4 oz. 96

baked, broiled, or microwaved, 4 oz. 124
Linguine:
dry, see "Pasta"
refrigerated, *(Contadina)*, 1¼ cups 240
refrigerated, plain or herb *(DiGiorno)*, 2.5 oz. 190
Linguine dishes, mix, garlic-butter
(Lipton Pasta & Sauce), 1 cup* 260
Liquor, pure distilled, unflavored (gin, scotch, etc.)
1 fl. oz.:
80 proof. 65
90 proof. 74
Liver:
beef, pan-fried, 4 oz. 246
chicken, simmered, 4 oz. 178
chicken, simmered, chopped, 1 cup 219
duck, raw, 1 oz. 39
goose, raw, 1 oz. 38
lamb, pan-fried, 4 oz. 270
turkey, simmered, 4 oz. 192
turkey, simmered, chopped, 1 cup 237
veal (calves), braised, 4 oz. 187
Liver cheese *(Oscar Mayer)*, 1.3-oz. slice 120
Liver pâté, see "Pâté"
Liverwurst (see also "Braunschweiger"), 2 oz.:
(Boar's Head Strassburger) 170
(Hansel 'n Gretel) 170
spread *(Underwood)* 170
Lo bok, see "Radish, Chinese"
Lobster, northern, meat only:
raw, 4 oz. 102
boiled or steamed, 4 oz. 111
boiled or steamed, 1 cup, 5.1 oz. 142
"Lobster," imitation, frozen or refrigerated:
chunk style *(Captain Jac Lobster Tasties)*, ½ cup 90
chunk style *(Louis Kemp Lobster Delights)*, ½ cup 80
salad *(Louis Kemp Lobster Delights)*, ½ cup 80
tail, whole *(Captain Jac Lobster Tasties)*, 4-oz. tail 120
Lobster, spiny, see "Spiny lobster"
Lobster sauce *(Progresso)*, ½ cup 100

Loganberries:
fresh, 1 cup 89
frozen, ½ cup 40
Long beans *(Frieda's)*, ¾ cup, 3 oz. 40
Long John Silver's:
entrees:
   clams, breaded, 2.5 oz. 250
   chicken plank, battered, 2-oz. piece 130
   fish, battered, 3.4-oz. piece 230
   fish, battered, jr. 2-oz. piece 140
   fish, lemon crumb, 2 pieces, 5.3 oz. 240
   fish, lemon crumb, a la carte, 2 pieces w/rice 480
   fish, lemon crumb, Add-a-Piece, 1 piece w/rice 150
   shrimp, battered, 1 piece 35
meal, lemon crumb fish 730
meals, everyday value:
   chicken plank, 2 pieces, w/fries 600
   chicken plank, 1 piece, w/3 shrimp, fries 550
   fish, jr., w/fries:
      2 pieces 620
      1 piece, w/chicken plank 610
      1 piece, w/3 shrimp 560
   shrimp, 5 pieces, w/fries 500
sandwiches, 1 piece:
   chicken, *Grab n Go* 330
   chicken, *Grab n Go* w/cheese 380
   fish, *Grab n Go* 340
   fish, *Grab n Go* w/cheese 390
   Ultimate Fish 430
   wrap, 12.5 oz. 840
salads:
   chicken, grilled 140
   garden 45
   ocean chef 130
   side 20
salad dressings, 1 pkt.:
   French or ranch, fat free 40
   Italian 90
   ranch 170
   Thousand Island 120

sides and soup:

broccoli cheese soup, 8-oz. bowl 180
cheese sticks, 5 pieces 160
coleslaw, 4 oz. 170
corn cobbette, plain, 1 piece 80
corn cobbette, w/butter, 1 piece 140
fries, regular, 3 oz. 250
fries, large, 5 oz. 420
hush puppy, 1 piece 60
rice, 4 oz. 180

sauces/condiments, 1 pkt.:

honey mustard 20
ketchup 10
malt vinegar 0
shrimp sauce 15
sweet 'n' sour sauce 20
tartar sauce 40

dessert pie, 1 piece:

chocolate creme 280
lemon, double 350
key lime creme cheese 310
pecan 390
pineapple creme cheesecake 310
strawberries n' creme 280

Loquat, 1 medium, .6 oz. 5
Lotus root:
(Frieda's), 1 cup, 3 oz. 50
boiled, drained, 4 oz. 75
Lotus seed:
raw, 1 oz. 25
dried, 1 oz. 94
Lunch combinations *(Lunchables),* 1 pkg.:
bologna/American 470
bologna/wild cherry 530
chicken/turkey deluxe 390
ham/cheddar 360
ham/punch 440
ham/Swiss 340
low fat, ham/*Surfer Cooler* 390
low fat, ham/punch 350

Lunch combinations *(cont.)*
low fat, turkey/*Pacific Cooler* 360
pizza, cheese, two 300
pizza, mozzarella/punch 450
pizza, pepperoni/mozzarella 330
pizza, pepperoni/orange 450
salami/American 430
turkey/cheddar 350
turkey/ham deluxe 370
turkey/Monterey jack 350
turkey/*Pacific Cooler* 450
turkey/*Surfer Cooler* 430
Lunch meat, loaf (see also specific listings), 2 oz.,
   except as noted:
(*Diet Delight* Deluxe) 160
barbecue *(Diet Delight)* 150
Dutch *(Diet Delight)* 160
honey *(Oscar Mayer)*, 1-oz. slice 35
Italian *(Diet Delight)* 150
old fashioned *(Oscar Mayer)*, 1-oz. slice 70
olive *(Boar's Head)* 130
olive *(Oscar Mayer)*, 1-oz. slice 70
pickle *(Diet Delight)* 110
pickle and pimiento *(Oscar Mayer)*, 1-oz. slice 80
pepper *(Diet Delight)* 110
spiced *(Oscar Mayer)*, 1-oz. slice 70
Lupin, boiled, ½ cup 98
Lychee, shelled:
raw, seeded, 1 oz. 19
dried, 1 oz. 79

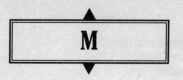

M

FOOD AND MEASURE	CALORIES

Macadamia nut:
(Mauna Loa), 1 oz. 220
dried, shelled, ½ cup 470
honey roasted *(Mauna Loa)*, 1 oz. 210
onion-garlic *(Mauna Loa)*, 1.4-oz. pkg. 320
Macaroni (see also "Pasta"):
uncooked, 2 oz. 211
cooked, elbow, 1 cup 197
cooked, small shells, 1 cup 162
cooked, spirals, 1 cup 189
cooked, vegetable (tri-color), 4 oz. 145
cooked, whole-wheat, 4 oz. 141
Macaroni entree, canned, and cheese
(Franco-American), 1 cup 210
Macaroni entree, frozen, 1 pkg., except as noted:
and beef *(Lean Cuisine)*, 10 oz. 270
and beef *(Stouffer's)*, 11½ oz. 420
and cheese *(Amy's)*, 9 oz. 390
and cheese *(Banquet)*, 9.5 oz. 320
and cheese *(Banquet* Family), 1 cup 210
and cheese *(Healthy Choice)*, 9 oz. 320
and cheese *(Kid Cuisine* Magical), 10.8 oz. 410
and cheese *(Lean Cuisine)*, 10 oz. 290
and cheese *(Marie Callender's)*, 13.5 oz. 510
and cheese *(Marie Callender's* Family), 1 cup 300
and cheese *(Stouffer's* 12 oz.), 1 cup or ½ pkg. 320
and cheese *(Stouffer's* 20 oz.), 1 cup 340
and cheese *(Stouffer's* 40 oz.), 1 cup 380
and cheese, nondairy *(Amy's* Soy Cheeze), 9 oz. 360
and cheese w/broccoli *(Stouffers)*, 10½ oz. 360
and cheese pot pie *(Banquet)*, 6.5 oz. 200
Macaroni entree mix, and cheese, dry:
(Kraft Deluxe Original), 3.5 oz. 320
(Kraft Original), 2.5 oz. 260

Macaroni entree mix *(cont.)*
(Kraft Thick'n Creamy), 2.5 oz. 260
w/white cheddar *(Kraft)*, 2.5 oz. 260
Mace, ground, 1 tsp. 8
Mackerel, meat only, 4 oz.:
Atlantic, raw 232
Atlantic, baked, broiled, or microwaved 297
king, raw 119
king, baked, broiled, or microwaved 152
Pacific and jack, raw 179
Pacific and jack, baked, broiled, or microwaved 228
Spanish, raw 158
Spanish, baked, broiled, or microwaved 179
Mackerel, canned, jack, boneless, drained, 4 oz. 177
Mackerel, smoked *(Spence & Co.)*, 2 oz. 180
Madras sauce, see "Curry sauce"
Mahi mahi, see "Dolphin fish"
Mai Tai mixer *(Trader Vic's)*, 4 fl. oz. 130
Malt coolers, *(Bartles & Jaymes)*, 12 fl. oz.:
original 190
berry or peach 210
berry, Brazilian Mist, or black cherry 200
Fuzzy Navel or tropical 230
kiwi strawberry 214
Margarita 260
Oriental dragon fruit 200
pina colada 270
strawberry daiquiri 220
Malted milk powder, 3 tbsp.:
natural *(Kraft* Instant) 90
chocolate *(Kraft* Instant) 80
Mammy apple, peeled, seeded, 1 oz. 14
Mandioca, see "Yuca"
Mango, fresh:
10.6-oz. fruit 135
peeled, sliced, ½ cup 54
Mango, dried:
(Frieda's), 4 pieces, 1.4 oz. 130
(Sonoma), 2 oz. 180

Mango drink *(Mango Mango!)*, 8 fl. oz. 130
Mango drink, mix* *(Tang)*, 8 fl. oz. 100
Mango-pineapple-banana smoothie *(Del Monte*
    Blenders), 6.25 fl. oz. 180
Manicotti entree, frozen, 1 pkg., except as noted:
cheese *(Stouffer's)*, 9 oz. 360
cheese *(Stouffer's)*, 1/12 of 61-oz. pkg. 160
cheese, three *(Healthy Choice)*, 11 oz. 300
cheese-spinach *(Lean Cuisine Hearty Portions)*, 15½ oz. . 370
Maple syrup, ¼ cup:
(Cary's/Maple Orchard's/MacDonald's Pure) 210
(Russell Farms) 200
Margarine, 1 tbsp., except as noted:
(Land O Lakes Stick/Tub) 100
(Land O Lakes Country Morning Blend Stick) 100
(Land O Lakes Country Morning Blend Tub) 80
(Nucoa No-Burn) 100
(Smart Balance) 80
light *(Land O Lakes* Country Morning Blend) 50
light *(Smart Balance)* 45
light *(Smart Beat* Trans-Fat Free) 20
light, unsalted *(Smart Beat)* 25
light, squeeze *(Smart Beat)* 5
soft *(Chiffon* Tub) 100
soft *(Parkay* Tub) 100
soft *(Parkay* Diet Tub) 50
spread *(Kraft Touch of Butter* Stick) 90
spread *(Kraft Touch of Butter* Tub) 60
spread *(Land O Lakes* Spread w/Sweet Cream Stick) 90
spread *(Land O Lakes* Spread w/Sweet Cream Tub) 80
spread *(Parkay* Stick 53%) 70
spread *(Parkay* Stick 70%) 90
spread *(Parkay Light* Tub 40%) 50
spread *(Parkay* Tub 50%) 60
squeeze *(Kraft Touch of Butter)* 80
squeeze *(Parkay* 64%) 80
whipped *(Chiffon)* 70
whipped *(Parkay)* 70
Margarita mixer, strawberry *(Trader Vic's)*, 4 fl. oz. 160

Marinade (see also "Stir-fry sauce" and specific sauce listings), 2 tbsp., except as noted:

citrus grill *(Lawry's* 30-Minute)	15
Hawaiian or hickory *(Lawry's* 30-Minute)	20
herb and garlic *(Lawry's* 30-Minute)	10
honey hickory *(World Harbors* Ember Wisp)	45
jerk *(Helen's Tropical Exotics),* 1 tbsp.	10
jerk, Caribbean *(Lawry's* 30-Minute)	25
lemon pepper *(Lawry's* 30-Minute)	10
lemon pepper and garlic *(World Harbors* Acadia)	35
mesquite *(Lawry's* 30-Minute)	5
red wine *(Lawry's* 30-Minute)	20
seasoned *(Lawry's),* 1 tbsp.	10
teriyaki *(Lawry's* 30-Minute)	25
Thai ginger *(Lawry's* 30-Minute)	10

Marjoram, dried, 1 tsp. 2
Marmalade, see "Jam and preserves"
Marrow beans, dried *(Frieda's),* ½ cup 120
Marrow squash, raw, trimmed, 1 oz. 4
Marshmallow, see "Candy"

Marshmallow topping, 2 tbsp.:

(Marshmallow Fluff)	60
(Smucker's)	120
creme *(Kraft)*	40

Mayonnaise, 1 tbsp.:

(Hellmann's/Best Foods)	100
(Kraft)	100
(Smart Beat Fat Free)	10
dressing *(Kraft* Fat Free)	10
dressing *(Kraft* Light)	50
dressing *(Miracle Whip)*	70
dressing *(Miracle Whip* Free)	15
dressing *(Miracle Whip* Light)	40
dressing *(Spin Blend)*	60
dressing *(Spin Blend* Fat Free)	15

McDonald's, 1 serving:

breakfast biscuit:

plain	290
bacon, egg, and cheese or sausage	470
sausage and egg	550

breakfast burrito 320
breakfast dishes:
    eggs, scrambled, 2 160
    hash browns 130
    hot cakes, plain 310
    hot cakes, w/syrup, margarine 570
    sausage 170
breakfast muffins:
    English 140
    Egg McMuffin 290
    Sausage McMuffin 360
    Sausage McMuffin w/egg 440
danish and muffin:
    apple bran muffin, lowfat 300
    apple danish 360
    cheese danish 410
    cinnamon roll 390
sandwiches:
    Arch Deluxe 550
    Arch Deluxe w/bacon 590
    Big Mac 560
    cheeseburger 320
    Crispy Chicken Deluxe 500
    Filet-O-Fish 450
    Fish Filet Deluxe 560
    Grilled Chicken Deluxe 440
    Grilled Chicken Deluxe, w/out mayo 300
    hamburger 260
    Quarter Pounder 420
    Quarter Pounder w/cheese 530
Chicken McNuggets:
    4 pieces 190
    6 pieces 290
    9 pieces 430
McNuggets sauce pkt.:
    barbeque or honey 45
    honey mustard or sweet and sour 50
    hot mustard 60
    mayonnaise, light 40

McDonald's *(cont.)*

fries:

small	210
large	450
Super Size	540

salads:

chicken, grilled	120
garden	35
croutons, 1 pkg.	50

salad dressing, 1 pkt.:

Caesar	160
ranch	230
red French, reduced calorie	160
vinaigrette, herb	50

desserts and shakes:

baked apple pie	260
chocolate chip cookie	170
McDonaldland Cookies, 1 pkg.	180
McFluffy, Butterfinger	620
McFluffy, M&M's or *Nestlé Crunch*	630
McFluffy, Oreo	570
shake, chocolate, strawberry, or vanilla, small	360
sundae, hot caramel	360
sundae, hot fudge	340
sundae, strawberry	290
sundae nuts	40
vanilla cone, reduced fat	150

Meat, see specific listings

"Meat," ground (see also " 'Burger,' vegetarian")
(Morningstar Farms Ground Meatless), ½ cup 60

Meat, lunch, see "Lunch meat" and specific listings

Meat loaf dinner, frozen, 1 pkg.:

(Banquet Extra Helping), 16 oz.	610
(Healthy Choice Traditional), 12 oz.	320

Meat loaf entree, frozen, 1 pkg.:

(Banquet Meal), 9.5 oz.	280
(Stouffer's Homestyle), 9⅞ oz.	390
in gravy *(Stouffer's),* ⅙ of 33-oz. pkg.	190

w/gravy, mashed potato:

(Marie Callender's), 14 oz.	540

(Marie Callender's Family), 1 patty, ½ cup potato . . . 300
(Stouffer's Hearty Portions), 17 oz. 480
gravy, savory, and *(Banquet* Family), 1 patty w/gravy . . . 190
w/whipped potato *(Lean Cuisine American Favorites),*
9⅜ oz. 250
w/whipped potato *(Stouffer's),* ⅙ of 69-oz. pkg. 380
"Meat" loaf mix, vegetarian *(Natural Touch),* 4 tbsp.
dry 100
Meat seasoning *(Aromat),* ¼ tsp. 0
Meat spread (see also specific listings) *(Oscar Mayer),*
2 oz. 130
Meat tenderizer, unseasoned *(Tone's),* 1 tsp. 7
"Meatball," vegetarian, w/gravy, canned
(Loma Linda Tender Rounds), 6 pieces 120
Meatball, refrigerated, w/barbecue sauce
(Lloyd's), 6 pieces, w/sauce 250
Meatball entree, frozen, 1 pkg.:
Italian style *(Healthy Choice Hearty Handfuls),* 6.1 oz. 320
Swedish *(Healthy Choice),* 9.1 oz. 280
Swedish *(Marie Callender's),* 12.5 oz. 520
Swedish *(Stouffer's),* 10¼ oz. 470
Swedish, w/pasta *(Lean Cuisine),* 9⅛ oz. 290
Meatball pocket, w/mozzarella, frozen *(Hot Pockets),*
4.5-oz. piece 320
Melon balls, frozen, cantaloupe/honeydew, ½ cup 28
Melon drink *(Mega Melon),* 8 fl. oz. 130
Mexican beans (see also "Chili beans"), canned,
½ cup:
(Allens/Brown Beauty Chili) 120
(El Rio) 110
(Old El Paso Mexe) 110
w/jalapeños *(Brown Beauty)* 120
w/jalapeños *(Trappey's* Mexi-Beans) 130
Mexican dinner (see also specific listings), frozen,
1 pkg.:
(Patio Fiesta), 12 oz. 350
(Patio Ranchers), 13 oz. 470
style *(Patio),* 13.25 oz. 470

Mexican dinner mix (see also specific listings), 2
   pieces*:
nacho cheese *(Old El Paso One Skillet Mexican* Kit) 490
salsa or taco *(Old El Paso One Skillet Mexican* Kit) 460
Milk, 8 fl. oz.:
buttermilk, cultured 99
buttermilk, light *(Friendship)* 120
whole, 3.3% fat 150
low fat, 2% fat 121
low fat, 2%, protein fortified 137
low fat, 1% fat 102
low fat, 1%, protein fortified 119
skim, nonfat 86
Milk, canned, 2 tbs.:
condensed, sweetened *(Carnation)* 130
evaporated *(Carnation)* 40
evaporated *(Carnation* Fat Free/Low Fat) 25
evaporated *(Pet)* 40
evaporated, filled *(Jerzee)* 35
evaporated, skim *(Jerzee)* 25
evaporated, skim *(Pet)* 25
Milk, chocolate, see "Chocolate milk"
Milk, dry:
buttermilk, sweet cream, 1 tbsp. 25
whole, 1 oz. 141
whole, 1/4 cup 159
nonfat *(Carnation),* 1/3 cup 80
nonfat, regular, 1 cup 435
nonfat, instant, 3.2-oz. pkt. 244
Milk, goat's, 1 cup 168
"Milk," nondairy (see also "Soy beverage"), 8 fl. oz.:
(Grainaissance Amazake Original) 150
(Rice Dream Original) 120
(Vitamite) 110
(Vitamite Nonfat) 90
flavored:
   (Grainaissance Amazake Gimme Green) 190
   almond shake, cocoa almond, hazelnut, sesame,
      vanilla pecan *(Grainaissance Amazake)* 200
   apricot or banana *(Grainaissance Amazake)* 160

carob *(Rice Dream)* 150
chocolate *(Rice Dream)* 170
coffee *(Grainaissance Amazake)* 170
mocha java *(Grainaissance Amazake)* 180
rice nog *(Grainaissance Amazake)* 190
vanilla *(Rice Dream)* 130
mix* *(Vitamite)* 110
mix*, chocolate *(Chocomite)* 120
Milk, sheep's, 1 cup 264
Milkfish, meat only:
raw, 4 oz. 168
baked, broiled, or microwaved, 4 oz. 215
Millet:
raw, 1 oz. 107
cooked, 4 oz. 135
hulled *(Arrowhead Mills),* ¼ cup 150
Millet flour *(Arrowhead Mills),* ¼ cup 110
Mincemeat, see "Pie filling"
Mint sauce *(Crosse & Blackwell),* 1 tsp. 5
Miso, soy, ½ cup 284
Mochi, plain *(Grainaissance* Organic), 1½ oz. . . . 110
Molasses, blackstrap *(New Morning),* 1 tbsp. 60
Monkfish, meat only:
raw, 4 oz. 86
baked, broiled, or microwaved, 4 oz. 110
Monosodium glutamate *(Tone's),* 1 tsp. 0
Mortadella, w/pistachos *(Boar's Head Cinghiale),* 2 oz. . 170
Mothbean, boiled, 4 oz. 133
Mother's loaf, pork, 1 oz. 80
Mousse mix, dry:
chocolate:
dark or milk *(Alsa),* 2 tbsp. 80
dark or milk *(Nestlé European Style),* ¼ pkg. 90
white *(Alsa),* 2 tbsp. 70
raspberry truffle *(Nestlé European Style),* ¼ pkg. . . . 90
Irish crème or mocha *(Nestlé European Style),* ¼ pkg. . . 90
Muffin, 1 piece, except as noted:
apple *(Awrey's),* 2½ oz. 250
apple or blueberry *(Awrey's),* 1½ oz. 130
banana, mini *(Awrey's),* 2 pieces, 1½ oz. 200

Muffin *(cont.)*

banana nut *(Awrey's Grande)*, 4 oz. 400
blueberry *(Awrey's Grande)*, 2½ oz. 340
blueberry *(Awrey's/Awrey's Muffin Top)*, 2½ oz. 210
blueberry *(Entenmann's)* 120
blueberry, mini *(Awrey's)*, 2 pieces, 1½ oz. 180
carrot raisin *(Awrey's Grande)*, 4 oz. 360
cheese streusel *(Awrey's Grande)*, 2½ oz. 380
chocolate chocolate chip *(Awrey's Grande)*, 2½ oz. 460
corn *(Awrey's)*, 1½ oz. 130
corn *(Awrey's)*, 2½ oz. 220
corn *(Entenmann's)* 210
cranberry nut *(Awrey's)* 120
English *(Awrey's)* 140
lemon poppyseed *(Awrey's)*, 1½ oz. 170
lemon poppyseed *(Awrey's Grande)*, 2½ oz. 390
lemon poppyseed mini *(Awrey's)*, 2 pieces, 1½ oz. 160
raisin bran *(Awrey's)*, 1½ oz. 110
raisin bran *(Awrey's Grande)*, 2½ oz. 340
raisin bran *(Awrey's/Awrey's Muffin Top)*, 2½ oz. 190

Muffin, frozen or refrigerated, 1 piece:

blueberry *(Sara Lee)* 220
corn *(Sara Lee)* 260

Muffin mix, 1 piece*, except as noted:

apple cinnamon *(Betty Crocker)* 170
apple cinnamon *(Pillsbury)* 180
apple cinnamon *(Sweet Rewards)* 140
apple streusel *(Betty Crocker)* 210
banana nut *(Betty Crocker Box/Pouch)* 170
banana nut *(Martha White)* 210
banana nut *(Pillsbury)* 170
blackberry *(Martha White/Mother's Best)* 170
blueberry *(Betty Crocker)* 160
blueberry *(Pillsbury)* 180
blueberry *(Pillsbury Low Fat)* 160
blueberry, wild *(Betty Crocker)* 170
blueberry, wild *(Sweet Rewards)* 120
bran *(Mother's Best)* 190
caramel nut *(Betty Crocker)* 170

chocolate, double *(Betty Crocker)* 200
chocolate chip *(Betty Crocker)* 170
chocolate chip *(Pillsbury)* 190
cinnamon *(Martha White)* 190
cinnamon *(Pillsbury)* 160
corn *(Betty Crocker)* 160
corn *(Gladiola)* 180
corn, yellow *(Martha White)* 180
honey bran *(Martha White)* 200
honey pecan *(Martha White)* 180
lemon poppyseed *(Betty Crocker* Box) 190
lemon poppyseed *(Betty Crocker* Pouch) 180
lemon poppyseed *(Martha White)* 210
oat bran *(Arrowhead Mills)*, dry, 1/3 cup 160
raspberry *(Martha White/Mother's Best)* 170
strawberry *(Martha White/Mother's Best)* 170
strawberry *(Pillsbury)* 180
whole grain *(Arrowhead Mills)*, dry, 1/3 cup 150
Mulberry:
10 berries, 1/2 oz. 7
1/2 cup 31
Mullet, striped, meat only:
raw, 4 oz. 133
baked, broiled, or microwaved, 4 oz. 170
Mung beans:
dry *(Arrowhead Mills)*, 1/4 cup 160
boiled, 1/2 cup 107
Mung beans, sprouted:
raw, 1 oz. 9
boiled, drained, 1/2 cup 13
Mungo beans, boiled, 1/2 cup 95
Mushroom, 1/2 cup:
fresh, raw, pieces 9
fresh, boiled, drained, pieces 21
canned, all styles *(BinB/Green Giant)* 30
canned, all styles w/garlic *(BinB)* 35
Mushroom, chanterelle, dried *(Frieda's)*, 2 pieces 15
Mushroom, enoki, fresh:
(Frieda's), 4 oz. 40

1 large, 4⅛″ long 2
Mushroom, morel, dried *(Frieda's)*, 3 pieces 15
Mushroom, oyster, fresh *(Frieda's)*, 3 oz. 20
Mushroom, padi straw, dried *(Frieda's)*, 6 pieces 15
Mushroom, porcini, dried *(Frieda's)*, 5 pieces 15
Mushroom, portobello, dried *(Frieda's)*, 7 pieces 5
Mushroom, shiitake:
fresh, raw *(Frieda's)*, 3 oz. 20
fresh, cooked, 4 medium or ½ cup pieces 40
dried, 4 medium, ½ oz. 44
frozen *(Seneca)*, ½ cup 20
Mushroom, wood ear, fresh *(Frieda's)*, 3 oz. 20
Mushroom blends:
pasta, soup, or steak *(Frieda's)*, 6 pieces 15
poultry, sauce, or stir-fry *(Frieda's)*, 4 pieces 15
Mushroom gravy, canned *(Franco-American)*, ¼ cup 20
Mussel, blue, meat only:
raw, 4 oz. 98
raw, 1 cup 129
boiled or steamed, 4 oz. 195
Mustard, prepared, 1 tsp., except as noted:
(Boar's Head Delicatessen Style) 0
(French's Classic Yellow) 0
(French's Hearty Deli) 5
(Kraft) 0
Dijon *(Grey Poupon)* 5
Dijon or honey *(French's)* 5
honey *(Boar's Head)* 10
w/horseradish *(French's)* 0
w/horseradish *(Kraft)* 0
hot *(Nance's)* 15
sweet onion *(French's)* 10
Mustard cabbage, see "Cabbage, mustard"
Mustard greens, ½ cup, except as noted:
fresh, chopped, raw, 1 oz. or ½ cup 7
fresh, chopped, boiled, drained 11
canned *(Allens Sunshine)* 30
Mustard powder, 1 tsp. 9
Mustard sauce *(Heluva* Good), 1 tsp. 6

Mustard seeds, 1 tsp. 15
Mustard spinach:
raw, chopped, ½ cup 17
boiled, drained, chopped, ½ cup 14
Mustard tallow, 1 tbsp. 115

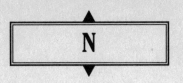

N

Nacho dip (see "Cheese dip")
Nacho snack, stuffed, frozen, 6 pieces:
(Totino's Grande) 210
cheese and beef, nacho, or taco *(Totino's)* 220
cheese, jalapeño *(Totino's)* 200
cheese, three *(Totino's)* 210
chicken and cheese *(Totino's)* 200
Name yam *(Frieda's),* 3 oz. 100
Natto, ½ cup 187
Navy bean, ½ cup:
dried, boiled 129
canned *(Allens)* 110
canned, w/bacon or bacon and jalapeño *(Trappey's)* 110
Navy bean, sprouted, raw, ½ cup 35
Nectarine:
1 medium, 2½″ diam. 67
sliced, ½ cup 34
New England sausage *(Oscar Mayer),* 2 slices,
 1.6 oz. 60
Noodle, Chinese:
cellophane or long rice, dry, 2 oz. 199
chow mein *(Frieda's),* 4 oz. 270
chow mein, ½ cup 119
Noodle, egg, dry, 2 oz., except as noted:
(Borden Enriched), 1 cup 210
(Kluski Enriched), 1 cup 220
(Manischewitz), 1¾ cup 210
fettuccine, plain or wheat *(Al Dente)* 220
linguine *(Al Dente)* 210
linguine, spinach *(Al Dente)* 220
spaetzel *(Maggi),* ⅙ pkg. 180
yolk-free *(Borden),* 1 cup 210
Noodle, egg, cooked:
1 cup 212

spinach, 1 cup 211
Noodle, egg-free, dry *(Borden* Eggless Enriched),
   2 oz. 210
Noodle, Japanese, dry, except as noted:
soba, cooked, 1 cup 113
somen, 2 oz. 203
somen, cooked, 1 cup 230
udon, cooked, 4 oz. 115
Noodle dinner, frozen, Asian stir-fry *(Amy's),* 10 oz. . . . 240
Noodle dishes, frozen, see "Noodle entree"
Noodle dishes, mix, 1 cup*:
Alfredo *(Lipton* Noodles & Sauce) 330
Alfredo, broccoli *(Lipton* Noodles & Sauce) 340
beef *(Lipton* Noodles & Sauce) 280
butter *(Lipton* Noodles & Sauce) 310
butter and herb *(Lipton* Noodles & Sauce) 300
cheddar cheese *(Kraft)* 430
chicken *(Kraft)* 330
chicken *(Lipton* Noodles & Sauce) 290
chicken, broccoli *(Lipton* Noodles & Sauce) 310
chicken, creamy *(Lipton* Noodles & Sauce) 320
chicken, sour cream-chives *(Lipton* Noodles &
   Sauce) 310
chicken Parmesan *(Lipton* Noodles & Sauce) 330
chicken Stroganoff *(Lipton* Noodles & Sauce) 300
chicken tetrazzini *(Lipton* Noodles & Sauce) 300
Noodle entree, frozen, 1 pkg., except as noted:
escalloped, and chicken *(Marie Callender's),* 1 cup 420
escalloped, and chicken *(Marie Callender's* Family),
   1 cup 260
Japanese noodles and vegetables *(Cascadian Farm*
   Veggie Bowl) 180
Romanoff *(Stouffer's),* ½ of 12-oz. pkg. 240
Nopales, see "Cactus leaves"
Nori, see "Seaweed"
Nut topping (see also specific listings)
Nutmeg, ground, 1 tsp. 12
Nuts, see specific listings

Nuts, mixed (see also "Snack mix"), 1 oz.:

w/peanuts *(River Queen* 70% Peanuts) 160
w/ or w/out peanuts *(River Queen)* 170
dry-roasted *(River Queen* Unsalted) 160
dry-roasted, w/peanuts 169
oil-roasted, w/peanuts 175

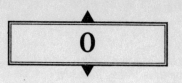

O

Oat (see also "Cereal"):
whole-grain, 1 oz. 110
flakes, rolled *(Arrowhead Mills)*, ⅓ cup 130
rolled or oatmeal, dry, 1 oz. 109
rolled or oatmeal, cooked, 1 cup 145
steel cut *(Arrowhead Mills)*, ¼ cup 170
Oat bran, dry *(Arrowhead Mills)*, ⅓ cup 150
Oat flour *(Arrowhead Mills)*, ⅓ cup 120
Oat groats *(Arrowhead Mills)*, ¼ cup 160
Ocean perch, Atlantic, meat only:
raw, 4 oz. 107
baked, broiled, or microwaved, 4 oz. 137
Ocean perch entree, frozen, breaded fillet
(Van de Kamp's), 2 pieces, 4 oz. 300
Octopus, meat only:
raw, 4 oz. 93
boiled or steamed, 4 oz. 186
Octopus, canned:
(Goya), ¼ cup 140
spiced, in red sauce *(Reese)*, 2 oz. 120
Oil, 1 tbsp.:
almond, canola, corn, cottonseed, olive, peanut, palm,
    safflower, sesame, sunflower, vegetable, walnut 120
(Arrowhead Mills Essential Balance Oil) 130
avocado or mustard 124
butter oil 112
coconut 117
cod liver, herring, salmon, or sardine 123
flax seed *(Arrowhead Mills)* 130
Okra, ½ cup, except as noted:
fresh, raw, sliced, ½ cup 19
fresh, boiled, drained, 8 pods, 3" × ⅝" 27
fresh, boiled drained, sliced 25
canned, cut *(Allens/Trappey's)* 25

Okra *(cont.)*

canned, gumbo *(Trappey's Creole)* 35
canned, w/tomatoes *(Allens/Trappey's)* 25
canned, w/tomatoes and corn *(Allens/Trappey's)* 30
frozen, boiled, drained, sliced, ½ cup 34

Old fashioned loaf, see "Lunch meat"

Olive, pickled, ½ oz., except as noted:
black, see "ripe," below
Calamata *(Krinos)*, 3 pieces 45
Calamata *(Zorba)*, 5 pieces, .5 oz. 90
Greek, black *(Zorba)*, 1 piece 60
green, w/pits, 10 small 33
green, w/pits, 10 large 45
green, w/pits, 10 giant 76
green, pitted, 1 oz. 33
green, Spanish *(Zorba)*, 2 pieces, .5 oz. 25
ripe, pitted:
    (Lindsay), 6 small, 5 medium, 4 large, or 1⅓ tbsp.
      chopped 25
    (Lindsay), 6 extra large, 1 colossal or 1 jumbo 25
    (Lindsay), 1 super colossal 15
    sliced *(Lindsay)*, 2 tbsp. 25
    wedged *(Lindsay)*, 2 tbsp. 30
ripe, w/pits *(Lindsay)*, 5 medium or 4 large 25
ripe, Greek, 10 medium 65
ripe, Greek, 10 extra large 89
stuffed w/almonds *(Reese)*, 4 pieces, .5 oz. 35
stuffed w/minced anchovies *(Reese)*, 4 pieces, .5 oz. 25

Olive Garden Garden Fare, 1 serving:
lunch entree:
    capellini pomodoro 380
    capellini primavera 350
    capellini primavera w/chicken 510
    chicken giardino 360
    linguine alla marinara 330
    shrimp primavera 410
minestrone soup, 6 fl. oz. 100
breadstick, plain, 1 piece 140
dinner entree:
    capellini pomodoro 620

capellini primavera 600
capellini primavera w/chicken 760
chicken giardino 550
grilled chicken Capri 550
linguine alla marinara 530
shrimp primavera 730
dessert, apple caramellina 570
Olive loaf, see "Lunch meat"
Olive oil, see "Oil"
Olive salad *(Progresso)*, 2 tbsp. 25
Omelet, see "Egg breakfast"
Ong choy, see "Spinach, water"
Onion, mature:
fresh, raw, chopped, ½ cup 30
fresh, raw, chopped, 1 tbsp. 4
fresh, boiled, drained, chopped, ½ cup 47
canned or in jars, whole *(Green Giant)*, ½ cup . . . 35
frozen *(Seneca)*, ⅔ cup 30
frozen rings, see "Onion rings"
Onion, boiler or Cipolline *(Frieda's)*, 3 pieces, 3 oz. 30
Onion, cocktail:
(Boar's Head Sweet Vidalia), 1 tbsp. 10
(Crosse & Blackwell), 1 tbsp. 0
Onion, dried:
flakes, 1 tbsp. 16
minced, 1 tsp. 7
Onion, french-fried, canned *(French's)*, 2 tbsp. . . . 45
Onion, green (scallion), raw, trimmed, w/top:
chopped, ½ cup 16
chopped, 1 tbsp. 2
Onion, Maui, fresh *(Frieda's)*, ⅓ cup, 3 oz. 10
Onion, pearl, fresh *(Frieda's)*, ⅔ cup, 3 oz. 30
Onion, pickled, sour *(London Pub)*, ¼ cup, 1.1 oz. 10
Onion, Welsh, 1 oz. 10
Onion dip, 2 tbsp.:
creamy *(Kraft Premium)* 45
French *(Breakstone's)* 50
French *(Frito-Lay)* 60
French *(Kraft)* 60
French *(Kraft Premium)* 50

Onion dip *(cont.)*
French *(Ruffles)* 70
French *(Ruffles* Lowfat) 40
green *(Kraft)* 60
toasted *(Breakstone's)* 50
Onion dip mix*, French *(Hidden Valley)*, 2 tbsp. 70
Onion flavor snack, 1 oz.:
(Funyons) 140
rings, *(Wise)* 140
Onion gravy, mix *(Loma Linda Gravy Quik)*, 1 tbsp. 20
Onion powder, 1 tsp. 10
Onion rings, frozen:
(Ore-Ida Classic/Gourmet), 4 rings 220
(Ore-Ida Onion Ringers), 6 rings 230
Onion salt *(Tone's)*, 1 tsp. 1
Opo squash *(Frieda's)*, 2/3 cup, 3 oz. 10
Opossum, meat only, roasted, 4 oz. 251
Orange:
blood *(Frieda's)*, 5 oz. 70
California navel:
    navel, 2$7/8$″ orange 65
    navel, sections w/out membrane, 1/2 cup 38
    Valencia, 2$5/8$″ orange 59
    Valencia, sections w/out membrane, 1/2 cup 44
Florida, 2$11/16$″ orange 69
Florida, sections w/out membrane, 1/2 cup 42
Orange, Mandarin, see "Tangerine"
Orange drink *(Snapple* Orangeade), 8 fl. oz. 120
Orange drink blends, 8 fl. oz., except as noted:
cranberry *(Tropicana Twister)* 120
cranberry *(Tropicana Twister* Light) 30
peach *(Tropicana Twister)* 120
peach strawberry *(Tropicana Twister)* 130
pineapple *(Tropicana)*, 11.5 fl. oz. 180
punch *(Kool-Aid Bursts)*, 6.75 fl. oz. 100
strawberry banana *(Tropicana Twister)* 130
strawberry banana *(Tropicana Twister* Light) 35
strawberry guava or raspberry *(Tropicana Twister)* 120
raspberry *(Tropicana Twister* Light) 35

Orange drink mix*, 8 fl. oz.:
(Kool-Aid) 100
(Kool-Aid Presweetened) 60
(Tang) 100
Orange juice, 8 fl. oz., except as noted:
fresh, 6 fl. oz. 83
(Hood) 120
(Minute Maid) 114
(Ocean Spray) 120
(Season's Best Regular/Homestyle/w/Calcium) 110
(Tropicana Pure Premium) 110
Orange juice blends, 8 fl. oz.:
(Minute Maid) 124
(Tropicana Bursters) 110
kiwi passion *(Tropicana Pure Tropics)* 100
peach mango *(Dole)* 120
peach mango *(Tropicana Pure Tropics)* 110
strawberry banana *(Chiquita* Cocktail) 120
strawberry banana *(Dole)* 120
strawberry banana *(Tropicana Pure Tropics)* 110
pineapple *(Season's Best)* 120
pineapple *(Tropicana Pure Tropics)* 110
Orange sauce, Oriental *(Ka•Me* Mandarin), 2 tbsp. 80
Oregano, dried, 1 tsp. 3
Oriental sauce, see "Stir-fry sauce" and specific
   listings
Oriental 5-spice *(Tone's)*, 1 tsp. 9
Oriental sauce, see specific listings
Oyster, meat only, 4 oz., except as noted:
Eastern:
   farmed, raw 67
   farmed, baked, broiled, or microwaved 90
   wild, raw, 6 medium, 3 oz. 57
   wild, baked, broiled, or microwaved 82
   wild, steamed or poached 155
Pacific, raw 93
Pacific, raw, boiled, or steamed, 1 medium 41
Pacific, boiled or steamed 185

Oyster, canned:
Eastern, wild, w/liquid, 4 oz. 78
Eastern, wild, w/liquid, 1 cup 170
Oyster plant, see "Salsify"
Oyster sauce, flavor *(Ka•Me),* 1 tbsp. 10
Oyster stew, see "Soup"

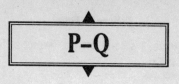

FOOD AND MEASURE   **CALORIES**

Pancake, frozen, 3 pieces, except as noted:
(Aunt Jemima Homestyle) 210
(Aunt Jemima Lowfat) 150
(Eggo) 270
blueberry or buttermilk *(Aunt Jemima)* 210
Pancake batter, frozen, ½ cup:
(Aunt Jemima Original) 250
blueberry *(Aunt Jemima)* 290
buttermilk *(Aunt Jemima)* 260
Pancake mix, ⅓ cup dry, except as noted:
(Betty Crocker Original Complete), ⅓ cup or 3 cakes* . . . 200
(Bisquick Shake 'N Pour Original), 3 cakes* 210
(Hungry Jack Original/*Extra Lights* Complete) 150
(Hungry Jack Extra Lights) 160
blue corn *(Arrowhead Mills)* 150
blueberry *(Bisquick Shake 'N Pour),* 3 cakes* 210
buttermilk *(Betty Crocker* Complete Box), ⅓ cup or 3
    cakes* 200
buttermilk *(Betty Crocker* Pouch) 180
buttermilk *(Betty Crocker* Pouch), 3 cakes* 230
buttermilk *(Bisquick Shake 'N Pour),* 3 cakes* 200
buttermilk *(Hungry Jack/Hungry Jack* Complete) 160
gluten-free or kamut *(Arrowhead Mills),* ¼ cup 130
oat bran or wild rice *(Arrowhead Mills)* 140
Pancake syrup (see also "Maple syrup"), ¼ cup:
(Country Kitchen Lite) 100
(Hungry Jack Lite) 100
regular or butter flavor *(Country Kitchen)* 200
regular or butter flavor *(Hungry Jack)* 210
Pancreas, braised:
beef, 4 oz. 307
veal (calf), 4 oz. 290

***Papa John's* Pizza**, 1 slice of 14″ pie, except as noted:
original crust pizza:

All the Meats	410
cheese	286
Garden Special	298
pepperoni	310
sausage	340
The Works	369

thin crust pizza:

All the Meats	330
cheese	220
Garden Special	238
pepperoni	266
sausage	270
The Works	319

sides:

breadstick, 1 piece	170
cheesesticks, 2 pieces	160
garlic sauce, 1 tbsp.	75
nacho cheese, 1 tbsp.	30
pizza sauce, 1 tbsp.	10

Papaya, fresh:

1-lb. fruit, 3½″ × 5⅛″	117
peeled, cubed, ½ cup	27
Paprika *(McCormick)*, ¼ tsp.	2

Parsley:

fresh, 10 sprigs	4
fresh, chopped, ½ cup	11
dried, 1 tsp.	1
Parsley root *(Frieda's)*, ⅔ cup, 3 oz.	10
Parsnip, boiled, drained, sliced, ½ cup	63
Passion fruit, fresh, purple, 1 medium	18

Passion fruit juice, fresh:

purple, 6 fl. oz.	95
yellow, 6 fl. oz.	111
Passion fruit juice drink *(Mauna La'i Paradise)*, 8 fl. oz.	130
Passion fruit syrup *(Trader Vic's)*, 1 fl. oz.	80

Pasta, dry (see also "Macaroni" and "Noodles"),
uncooked, 2 oz., except as noted:

all styles *(Contadina)*	210

all styles *(Delverde)* 200
angel hair, rigatoni, or rotini *(Al Dente Selecta)* 200
elbow style *(DeBoles),* ¼ pkg. 200
elbow style w/corn *(DeBoles),* ⅙ pkg. 200
w/egg, see "Noodles, egg"
fettuccine, all varieties *(DeBoles),* ¼ pkg. 200
fettuccine, garlic, roasted *(Al Dente Selecta)* 220
fettuccine, w/Jerusalem artichoke or rice *(DeBoles)* 210
lasagna or ribbon *(DeBoles),* ¼ pkg. 200
linguine, spaghetti, or ziti *(DeBoles)* 210
penne *(DeBoles)* 210
penne or rigatoni, garlic-parsley or tomato-basil
    (DeBoles), ¼ pkg. 200
penne or spirals, w/rice *(DeBoles),* ¼ pkg. 210
ribbon, regular or whole wheat *(DeBoles)* 210
rigatoni *(DeBoles)* 210
rotelle, roasted garlic and herb *(Mueller's)* 210
rotelle, tricolor *(Contadina)* 210
rotini *(DeBoles),* ¼ pkg. 200
rotini, garlic-parsley, primavera, or tomato-basil
    (DeBoles) 210
shells *(DeBoles),* ¼ pkg. 200
spaghetti, w/corn garlic-parsley, spinach, or tomato-
    basil *(DeBoles),* ¼ pkg. 200
spaghetti, w/Jerusalem artichoke or rice *(DeBoles),*
    ¼ pkg. 210
tricolor *(Borden)* 210
whole wheat, all styles, except ribbon *(DeBoles)* 210
Pasta, cooked, 1 cup:
plain 197
spinach 183
whole wheat 174
Pasta, refrigerated, see specific pasta listings
Pasta dinner, frozen (see also specific pasta listings),
    w/beef and broccoli *(Marie Callender's),* 15-oz. pkg. . 570
Pasta dishes, frozen (see also "Pasta entree, frozen"):
Alfredo *(Green Giant Pasta Accents),* 2 cups 210
cheddar, creamy *(Green Giant Pasta Accents),* 2⅓ cups . 250
cheddar, white *(Green Giant Pasta Accents),* 1¾ cups . . . 270
Florentine *(Green Giant Pasta Accents),* 2 cups 310

Pasta dishes, frozen *(cont.)*

garden herb seasoning *(Green Giant Pasta Accents)*,
  2 cups 230
garlic or lasagna *(Green Giant Pasta Accents)*, 2 cups . . . 260
marinara *(Cascadian Farm Veggie Bowl)*, 9-oz. pkg. 180
Oriental style *(Green Giant Pasta Accents)*, 2½ cups 260
primavera *(Cascadian Farm Veggie Bowl)*, 9-oz. pkg. . . . 270
primavera *(Green Giant Pasta Accents)*, 2¼ cups 290
Pasta dishes, mix (see also specific pasta listings),
  1 cup*, except as noted:
butter and herb *(Lipton Pasta & Sauce)* 270
cheddar broccoli *(Lipton Pasta & Sauce)* 340
cheddar cheese, mild *(Lipton Pasta & Sauce)* 290
chicken herb Parmesan *(Lipton Pasta & Sauce)* 280
chicken stir-fry *(Lipton Pasta & Sauce)* 270
garlic, creamy *(Lipton Pasta & Sauce)* 350
garlic, roasted, chicken *(Lipton Pasta & Sauce)* 290
garlic, roasted, and olive oil w/tomato *(Lipton Pasta &*
  Sauce) 270
hamburger, see "Hamburger entree mix"
herb, savory, w/garlic *(Lipton Pasta & Sauce)* 280
mushroom, creamy *(Lipton Pasta & Sauce)* 320
salad, ¾ cup*:
  Caesar *(Suddenly Salad)* 220
  Caesar *(Suddenly Salad Low Fat)* 170
  Caesar, creamy *(Kraft)* 350
  classic *(Suddenly Salad)* 250
  classic *(Suddenly Salad Lower Fat)* 210
  garden, Italian *(Suddenly Salad)* 140
  garden primavera *(Kraft)* 280
  Italian *(Kraft Light)* 190
  Parmesan peppercorn *(Kraft)* 360
  ranch and bacon *(Kraft)* 360
  ranch and bacon *(Suddenly Salad)* 330
  ranch and bacon *(Suddenly Salad Low Fat)* 180
spicy Thai *(Fantastic Foods Ready, Set, Pasta! Cup)*,
  1 pkg. 200
Pasta entree, canned (see also specific listings), 1 cup:
w/meat sauce, twists *(Franco-American Superiore)* 250
w/meatballs in tomato sauce *(Franco-American Garfield)* . 260

Pasta entree, frozen (see also "Pasta dishes, frozen" and specific pasta listings), 1 pkg., except as noted:

Alfredo, primavera *(Lean Cuisine)*, 10 oz. 290
cheddar, w/beef and tomatoes *(Stouffer's)*, 11 oz. 500
w/cheddar and broccoli *(Banquet)*, 9.5 oz. 330
w/Italian sausage *(Banquet Family)*, 1 cup 340
w/Italian sausage and peppers *(Banquet)*, 9.5 oz. 300
primavera *(Amy's)*, 9.5 oz. 320
stuffed, trio *(Marie Callender's)*, 10.5 oz. 380
vegetable Italiano *(Healthy Choice)*, 10 oz. 240

Pasta flour, see "Semolina flour"

Pasta salad, see "Pasta dishes, mix"

Pasta sauce, tomato (see also "Tomato sauce" and specific sauce listings), ½ cup:

(Muir Glen Chunky) 80
(Prego Extra Chunky Tomato Supreme) 130
(Prego No Salt) 110
(Prego Traditional) 140
(Progresso Spaghetti) 100
(Ragú Old World Traditional) 80
w/basil *(Classico* Di Napoli) 50
w/basil *(Prego)* 110
w/basil *(Ragu* Light No Sugar) 60
w/basil, summer *(Five Brothers)* 60
w/beef, ground *(Aunt Millie's* Chunky) 100
w/beef, sauteed *(Ragú* Hearty) 120
cheese, see "Cheese sauce, cooking"
w/cheese, four *(Classico* Di Parma) 80
w/cheese, three *(Prego)* 100
w/eggplant, grilled, w/Parmesan *(Five Brothers)* 100
garden combination *(Prego* Extra Chunky) 100
garden combination *(Ragú* Chunky Garden) 110
garden combination, chunky *(Ragú* Light) 50
w/garlic *(Prego* Extra Chunky Supreme) 140
w/garlic, Parmesan *(Prego* Extra Chunky) 120
w/garlic, roasted *(Classico* Di Sorrento) 60
w/garlic, roasted *(Ragú* Hearty) 120
w/garlic, roasted, and herb *(Prego)* 110
w/garlic, roasted, or garlic and onion *(Muir Glen)* 50

Pasta sauce *(cont.)*

w/garlic and onion *(Ragú Chunky Garden)* 120
w/garlic, oven roasted, and onion *(Five Brothers)* 70
w/green pepper and mushroom *(Muir Glen)* 70
hamburger *(Prego)* 120
w/herbs *(Ragú Hearty)* 110
w/herbs, Italian *(Muir Glen)* 60
w/herbs and olive oil *(Ragú Pasta Toss)* 120
Italian, cooking *(Ragú Traditional)* 60
leek and sun-dried tomato *(Al Dente Luscious)* 100
marinara *(Aunt Millie's Traditional)* 70
marinara *(Prego)* 110
marinara *(Prince Chunky)* 70
marinara *(Ragú Old World)* 80
marinara, cabernet *(Muir Glen)* 50
marinara, w/pizza paste *(Aunt Millie's)* 70
marinara or mushroom *(Prince Traditional)* 50
w/meat/meat flavor:
    (Aunt Millie's Traditional) 80
    (Prego) 140
    (Prince Chunky) 90
    (Prince Traditional) 50
    (Progresso) 100
    (Ragú Old World) 80
w/mushroom:
    (Prego Extra Chunky Supreme) 130
    (Prego Made With Mushrooms) 150
    (Prince Chunky) 70
    (Ragú Old World) 80
    and diced tomatoes *(Prego Extra Chunky)* 110
    w/extra spice or green pepper *(Prego Extra Chunky)* . 120
    and garlic *(Prego)* 110
    and garlic, chunky *(Ragú Light)* 50
    and green pepper *(Ragú Chunky Garden)* 110
    and herb *(Muir Glen)* 45
    and olives *(Classico Di Sicilia)* 70
    and onion *(Ragú Chunky Garden)* 120
    portabello *(Classico Di Toscana)* 70
    portabello *(Muir Glen)* 60
    sauteed *(Five Brothers)* 70

super *(Ragú* Chunky Garden) 120
olive and caper *(Al Dente* Outrageous) 90
w/olive and garlic *(Ragú* Chunky Garden) 120
w/onion and garlic *(Prego* Extra Chunky) 110
w/onion and garlic diced *(Prego)* 120
w/onion and garlic sauteed *(Ragú* Hearty) 120
w/onion and mushroom *(Ragú* Hearty) 110
w/Parmesan *(Prego)* 140
w/Parmesan and Romano *(Ragú* Hearty) 120
peccorino, romano & herb *(Classico* Di Palermo) 80
w/peppers and onions *(Classico* Di Salerno) 60
w/pepperoni *(Prego)* 120
w/red pepper, roasted *(Muir Glen)* 60
w/red pepper, roasted, and garlic *(Five Brothers)* 90
w/red pepper, roasted, and garlic *(Prego)* 110
w/red pepper, roasted, and onion *(Ragú* Chunky
    Garden) 120
w/red pepper, spicy *(Classico* Di Roma Arrabbiata) 60
w/red pepper, spicy *(Ragú* Hearty) 110
w/red wine and herbs *(Ragú* Hearty) 100
Romano *(Muir Glen)* 90
Romano w/garlic *(Five Brothers)* 90
w/sausage, Italian and fennel *(Classico* D'Abruzzi) 90
w/sausage, Italian, and garlic *(Prego)* 120
spinach and cheese Florentine *(Classico* Di Firenze) 80
w/spinach and cheese *(Ragú* Chunky Garden) 120
sun-dried tomato *(Muir Glen)* 45
sun-dried tomato and olives *(Classico* Di Capri) 80
w/sweet pepper and onion *(Muir Glen)* 40
w/sweet pepper and *(Ragú* Chunky Garden) 110
tomato, Alfredo *(Classico* Di Liguria) 120
tomato, Alfredo *(Five Brothers)* 150
tomato, fire-roasted, and garlic *(Classico* Di Siena) 60
tomato, Mediterranean, roasted *(Five Brothers)* 90
tomato, spicy, and pesto *(Classico* Di Genoa) 90
w/vegetables *(Prego* Extra Chunky Supreme) 120
w/vegetables, garden *(Muir Glen)* 60
w/vegetables, garden, primavera *(Five Brothers)* 70
w/vegetables, super, primavera *(Ragú* Chunky Garden) . . 110

Pasta sauce, refrigerated, tomato, ½ cup, except as noted:

cheese, four *(Di Giorno),* ¼ cup 200
marinara *(Contadina)* 80
marinara *(Di Giorno)* 100
marinara, mushroom *(Contadina)* 70
marinara, garlic, roasted *(Contadina)* 60
meat *(Di Giorno* Traditional) 120
olive oil-garlic, w/cheeses *(Di Giorno),* ¼ cup 370
tomato, chunky, w/basil *(Di Giorno Light Varieties)* 70
tomato, herb Parmesan *(Contadina)* 140
tomato, plum, and mushroom *(Di Giorno)* 70
vegetable, garden *(Contadina)* 40

Pastrami, 2 oz.:

(Boar's Head First Cut) 90
(Boar's Head Round) 70
(Healthy Choice) 60
(Healthy Deli) 80
turkey, see "Turkey pastrami"

Pastry, see specific listings

Pastry shell (see also "Pie crust"):

patty *(Pepperidge Farms),* 1 shell 230
puff, sheet *(Pepperidge Farms),* ⅛ sheet 200
tart *(Oronoque),* 3″ shell 140
tart *(Pet-Ritz),* 3″ shell 130

Pastry filling (see also "Pie filling"), canned, 2 tbsp.:

all fruits, except date, prune plum, and strawberry
    (Solo) 80
almond *(Solo)* 120
date *(Solo)* 100
nut, fancy *(Solo)* 140
pecan *(Solo)* 130
poppy seed *(Solo)* 140
prune plum or strawberry *(Solo)* 70

Pâté, canned (see also "Liverwurst"):

chicken liver, 1 oz. 57
chicken liver, 1 tbsp. 26
goose liver, smoked, 1 oz. 131
goose liver, smoked, 1 tbsp. 60

Pâté de Campagne *(Charcuterie de Bretagne),* 2 oz. 200

Pea pod, Chinese, see "Peas, edible-podded"
Peach:
fresh, 2½″ peach, 4 per lb. 37
fresh, sliced, ½ cup 37
canned, see "Peach, canned"
dried, sulfured, halves, ½ cup 192
dried, sulfured, 10 halves, 4.6 oz. 311
frozen, sliced, sweetened, ½ cup 118
Peach, canned, halves or slices, ½ cup, except as
  noted:
in juice *(Del Monte* Fruit Naturals) 60
in juice *(Del Monte* Fruit Naturals Cup), 4 oz. 50
in extra light syrup *(Del Monte* Lite Cling/Freestone) 60
in extra light syrup *(Del Monte* Lite Cup), 4 oz. 50
in light syrup *(Del Monte* Orchard Select) 80
in heavy syrup *(Del Monte/Del Monte* Melba/Whole
  Spiced) 100
in heavy syrup diced *(Del Monte* Cup), 4 oz. 80
raspberry flavor, natural *(Del Monte)* 80
spice *(Del Monte* Natural Harvest) 80
Peach butter *(Smucker's),* 1 tbsp. 45
Peach drink *(Fruitopia* Peachberry Quencher), 8 fl. oz. . . . 112
Peach juice blend *(Dole* Orchard), 8 fl. oz. 140
Peach nectar *(R. W. Knudsen),* 8 fl. oz. 120
Peach-raspberry smoothie *(Del Monte* Blenders),
  6.25 fl. oz. 200
Peanut, shelled:
(Beer Nuts Classic), 1 oz. 170
(Beer Nuts Old Fashioned), 1 oz. 185
(River Queen Salted), 3 tbsp. or 1 oz. 150
(River Queen Unsalted), 3 tbsp. or 1 oz. 160
Cajun *(River Queen),* 3 tbsp., .9 oz. 150
dry-roasted *(Arrowhead Mills* Valencia), ¼ cup 190
dry-roasted *(Frito-Lay),* 1.1 oz. 200
dry-roasted *(River Queen),* 1 oz. 160
honey mustard *(Beer Nuts),* ¼ cup, .9 oz. 140
honey-roasted *(Frito-Lay),* 1.6 oz. 270
honey-roasted *(River Queen),* 3 tbsp., .9 oz. 150
hot *(Beer Nuts* Cajun Devil), ¼ cup, .9 oz. 140
hot *(Frito-Lay),* 1.1 oz. 190

Peanut *(cont.)*
w/sesame seeds *(Beer Nuts)*, ¼ cup, .9 oz. 130
Spanish *(River Queen)*, 3 tbsp., 1 oz. 150
sweetened, salted *(River Queen* Pub Nuts)*, ¼ cup,
  1.2 oz. 190
Peanut butter, chunky or creamy, 2 tbsp.:
(Arrowhead Mills/Arrowhead Mills Easy Spread) 200
(Jif/Jif Reduced Fat) 190
(Laura Scudder's Old Fashioned/Reduced Fat) 200
(Smucker's Natural/Reduced Fat) 200
(Teddie/Teddie Old Fashioned/25% Less Fat) 190
Peanut topping (see also specific listings), 2 tbsp.:
(Teddie) 200
peanut butter caramel *(Smucker's)* 150
Peanut butter and jelly *(Goober's)*, 3 tbsp. 230
Peanut sauce, Oriental, Thai satay *(Ka•Me)*, 2 tbsp. 80
Pear:
fresh, w/peel, Bartlett, 1 medium, 2½ per lb. 98
fresh, sliced, ½ cup 49
fresh, Asian, dried, 2 oz. 149
dried, halves, ½ cup 236
Pear, canned, halves or slices, ½ cup, except as noted:
in juice *(Del Monte* Fruit Naturals) 60
in extra light syrup *(Del Monte* Lite) 60
in extra light syrup *(Del Monte* Lite Cup), 4 oz. 50
in light syrup, Bartlett *(Del Monte* Orchard Select) 80
in heavy syrup *(Del Monte)* 100
in heavy syrup diced *(Del Monte* Cup), 4 oz. 80
ginger flavor, natural *(Del Monte)* 90
Pear juice *(Heinke's/R.W. Knudsen* Organic), 8 fl. oz. . . . 120
Pear nectar *(Santa Cruz)*, 8 fl. oz. 120
Peas, see specific listings
Peas, cream, canned *(East Texas Fair)*, ½ cup 100
Peas, crowder *(Allens/East Texas Fair/Homefolks)*,
  ½ cup 110
Peas, edible-podded:
fresh, raw *(Frieda's* Snow), 1 cup, 3 oz. 35
fresh, raw *(Frieda's* Sugar Snap), ⅔ cup, 3 oz. 35
fresh, boiled, drained, ½ cup 34
frozen *(Green Giant* Sugar Snap), ¾ cup 35

frozen *(Green Giant Harvest Fresh* Sugar Snap), ⅔ cup . . 50
frozen *(Seneca* Snap), ⅔ cup 45
frozen, boiled, drained, ½ cup 42
Peas, field, canned, ½ cup:
fresh shell *(Sunshine)* 120
fresh shell w/snaps *(Allens/East Texas Fair/Homefolks)* . . 120
dry, w/bacon *(Trappey's)* 90
dry, w/bacon and snaps *(Trappey's)* 110
Peas, green, sweet, fresh:
raw, in pod, 1 lb. 140
raw, shelled, ½ cup 58
boiled, drained, ½ cup 67
Peas, green, canned, ½ cup:
(Del Monte/Del Monte No Salt) 60
(Seneca/Seneca No Salt) 70
early or sweet *(Green Giant/Green Giant* 50% Less
  Sodium) 60
early or sweet *(LeSueur)* 60
very young, small *(Del Monte)* 60
Peas, green, dried *(Frieda's)*, ⅓ cup, 3 oz. 130
Peas, green, frozen, ⅔ cup, except as noted:
(Seneca) 80
baby, early *(Green Giant Harvest Fresh LeSueur)* 70
early June *(LeSueur)* 60
garden *(Cascadian Farm)* 70
sweet *(Green Giant)* 70
sweet *(Green Giant Harvest Fresh)* 60
sweet, baby *(LeSueur Harvest Fresh)* 70
tiny *(John Cope's)* 70
tiny *(Seabrook)* 70
in butter sauce, baby, early *(LeSueur)*, ¾ cup 100
in butter sauce, sweet *(Green Giant)*, ¾ cup 100
Peas, green, combinations:
canned, w/carrots *(Del Monte)*, ½ cup 60
canned, w/carrots *(Green Giant)*, ½ cup 50
canned, w/carrots *(Seneca)*, ½ cup 60
canned, w/mushrooms and onions *(LeSueur)*, ½ cup 60
canned, w/pearl onions *(Green Giant)*, ½ cup 60
frozen, w/carrots *(Cascadian Farm)*, ⅔ cup 50
frozen, w/carrots *(Seneca)*, ⅔ cup 50

Peas, green, combinations *(cont.)*
frozen, w/mushrooms *(LeSueur)*, ¾ cup 60
frozen, w/onions *(Seneca)*, ⅔ cup 70
frozen, w/pearl onions *(Cascadian Farm)*, ¾ cup 60
frozen, w/pearl onions *(Green Giant)*, ⅔ cup . . . . ⌐. . . 60
frozen, w/pearl onions *(Green Giant Harvest Fresh)*,
   ½ cup 50
Peas, lady, canned, ½ cup:
(Sunshine) 100
w/snaps *(East Texas Fair)* 100
Peas, pepper, canned *(East Texas Fair)*, ½ cup 120
Peas, purple hull, canned *(Allens/East Texas Fair/*
   Homefolks), ½ cup 120
Peas, snow or sugar snap, see "Peas, edible-podded"
Peas, split, see "Split peas"
Peas, sprouted, raw, ½ cup 77
Peas, sweet, see "Peas, green"
Peas, white acre, canned *(East Texas Fair)*, ½ cup 100
Peas, and carrots or onions, see "Peas, green,
   combinations"
Pecan, shelled:
dried, 1 oz. 190
dried, halves, ⅓ cup 240
dry-roasted, 1 oz. 187
oil-roasted, 1 oz. 195
Pecan filling, see "Pastry filling"
Pecan flour, 1 oz. 93
Pecan topping, 2 tbsp.:
praline sauce *(Trader Vic's)* 120
in syrup *(Smucker's)* 170
Pectin, see "Fruit pectin"
Penne, plain, see "Pasta"
Penne dishes, mix, dry:
Alfredo sauce *(Annie's)*, ⅔ cup 270
w/spicy sauce *(Al Dente)*, ½ cup 240
tomato marinara *(Fantastic Foods Healthy*
   Complements), ½ cup 200
Penne entree, frozen, 1 pkg.:
and pepperoni *(Marie Callender's)*, 15 oz. 800
w/tomato sauce *(Healthy Choice)*, 8 oz. 230

w/tomato sauce basil *(Lean Cuisine)*, 10 oz. 270
Pepper, seasoning:
black, red or cayenne, ground, 1 tsp. 6
chili, 1 tsp. 9
seasoned *(Lawry's)*, ¼ tsp. 0
white, 1 tsp. 7
Pepper, banana, hot or mild *(Vlasic)*, 1 oz. 5
Pepper, bell, see "Pepper, sweet"
Pepper, cherry:
(Progresso Hot), 1-oz. piece 10
(Progresso So Hot/Sliced), 2 tbsp. 25
Pepper, chili, fresh:
all varieties *(Frieda's* Cucina), 1-oz. pepper 10
green and red, 1 medium, 1.6 oz. 18
green and red, chopped, ½ cup 30
Pepper, chili, in jars:
chopped, w/liquid, ½ cup 17
green, whole *(Old El Paso* Peeled), 1 piece 10
green, chopped *(Old El Paso)*, 2 tbsp. 5
green, diced *(Pancho Villa)*, 2 tbsp. 5
Pepper, chili, relish, pickle *(Patak's)*, 1 tbsp. 45
Pepper, jalapeño:
(La Victoria Marinated/Pickled), 1.1 oz. 10
whole *(Old El Paso* Peeled), 2 pieces 5
whole *(Old El Paso* Pickled), 3 pieces 5
diced *(La Victoria)*, 1.1 oz. 10
diced, hot *(Vlasic)*, 1 oz. 10
sliced *(La Victoria* Nacho), 1.1 oz. 0
sliced *(Old El Paso)*, 2 tbsp. 10
Pepper, roasted, see "Pepper, sweet, in jars"
Pepper, stuffed, entree, frozen:
(Stouffer's), 10 oz. 200
(Stouffer's), ½ of 15½-oz. pkg. 180
(Stouffer's), ¼ of 32-oz. pkg. 190
Pepper, sweet:
fresh, green and red, raw, 1 medium, 3¾" × 3" 20
fresh, green and red, raw, chopped, ½ cup 13
fresh, green and red, boiled, drained, 1 medium 20
fresh, yellow, raw, 1 large, 5" × 3" 50
fresh, yellow, raw, 10 strips, 1.8 oz. 14

Pepper, sweet *(cont.)*
freeze-dried, 1 tbsp. 1
frozen, red *(Seneca)*, ¾ cup 25
Pepper, sweet, in jars:
fried w/onions *(Progresso)*, 2 tbsp. 20
roasted *(Progresso)*, 2 pieces, 1 oz. 10
roasted, fire, w/garlic, oil *(Paesana)*, 2 tbsp. 20
salad, w/oregano, garlic *(B&G)*, 1 oz. 10
Pepper, sweet, marinated, sun-dried, in jars
(Antica Italia), 1 oz. 170
Pepper salad:
(B&G), 1 oz. 10
drained *(Progresso)*, 2 tbsp. 15
Pepper sauce (see also specific listings), hot, 1 tsp.,
   except as noted:
(Frank's Red Hot) 0
(Louisiana) 0
(Tabasco/Tabasco Garlic) 0
balsamic *(Roland)*, 1 tbsp. 10
habanero *(Tabasco)* 5
jalapeño *(Tabasco)*, 3.5 oz. 15
Pepper steak, see "Beef entree"
Pepperoncini:
(Progresso Tuscan), 3 pieces, 1 oz. 10
(Zorba), 5 pieces, 1.1 oz. 15
Pepperoni *(Oscar Mayer)*, 15 slices, 1.1 oz. 140
Perch (see also "Ocean perch"), meat only:
raw, 4 oz. 103
baked, broiled, or microwaved, 4 oz. 133
Persimmon, fresh:
(Frieda's), 5 oz. 100
Japanese, 1 medium 118
native, 1 medium, 1.1 oz. 32
Persimmon, dried:
(Frieda's Fuyu), ⅓ cup, 1.4 oz. 140
Japanese, 1 oz. 78
Pesto sauce, ¼ cup, except as noted:
(Sonoma) 110
creamy *(Five Brothers)* 110
Genovese *(Italia In Talola)*, 2 tbsp. 160

refrigerated *(Di Giorno)* 320
refrigerated, w/basil *(Contadina)* 290
refrigerated, w/basil *(Contadina* Reduced Fat) 230
refrigerated, basil and garlic *(Christopher Ranch)* 230
refrigerated, w/sun-dried tomato *(Contadina)* 250
Pheasant, raw:
meat w/skin, 4 oz. 205
meat only, 4 oz. 151
meat only, ½ breast, 6.4 oz. 243
Picante sauce (see also "Salsa"), 2 tbsp.:
all styles *(Muir Glen)* 10
all styles *(Pace)* 10
cheese, see "Cheese sauce"
hot *(Old El Paso* Thick 'n Chunky) 10
medium *(Old El Paso* Thick 'n Chunky) 10
mild *(Old El Paso* Thick 'n Chunky) 10
Pickle, cucumber, 1 oz., except as noted:
bread and butter *(Claussen),* 4 slices, 1 oz. 20
bread and butter *(Claussen* Sandwich), 2 slices, 1.2 oz. . . 25
bread and butter *(Mrs. Fanning's),* 3 pieces or 1 oz. 25
bread and butter midgets *(Vlasic* Milwaukee) 40
chips, w/honey *(Pickle Eater's),* about 6 pieces, 1 oz. 25
cornichons *(Italica),* 7 piecos, 1.1 oz. 0
dill, baby *(Pickle Eater's)* 0
dill, garlic *(Ba-Tampte)* 0
dill, halves *(Del Monte),* ¼ pickle, 1 oz. 5
dill, hamburger chips *(Del Monte),* 5½ chips 5
dill, whole *(Del Monte),* 1½ pieces, 1 oz. 5
dill, kosher *(Pickle Eater's* Deli) 0
dill, kosher, chips *(Claussen),* 4 chips, 1 oz. 5
dill, kosher, mini *(Claussen),* 8-oz. piece 5
dill, kosher, spears *(Pickle Eater's)* 0
dill, kosher, whole, tiny *(Del Monte),* 1½ pieces, 1 oz. 5
dill, Polish, spears *(Vlasic)* 5
garlic, hearty *(Claussen* Deli Style), ½ piece, 1 oz. 5
sour, half *(Ba-Tampte)* 0
sour, half *(Claussen)* 5
sweet, all varieties *(Del Monte)* 40
sweet, all varieties *(Vlasic)* 40
Pickle loaf, see "Lunch meat loaf"

Pickle relish, cucumber (see also specific listings), 1 tbsp.:

(Crosse & Blackwell Branston)	25
dill, chunky *(Nalley)*	0
hamburger *(Del Monte)*	20
hamburger *(Nalley)*	15
hot dog *(Del Monte)*	15
hot dog *(Nalley)*	15
piccalilli, tomato *(Pickle Eater's)*	10
red hot *(Ron's)*	15
sweet *(Del Monte)*	20
sweet, honey *(Pickle Eater's)*	15
sweet, regular or curry flavor *(Vlasic)*	15
Pickling spice *(Tone's),* 1 tsp.	10

Pie:

apple *(Entenmann's* Homestyle), 1/6 pie	340
coconut custard *(Entenmann's),* 1/5 pie	340
pecan *(Entenmann's),* 1/5 pie	550
pumpkin, custard *(Entenmann's),* 1/5 pie	310

Pie, frozen, (see also "Cobbler"):

apple:

(Amy's), 4 oz.	220
(Mrs. Smith's), 1/8 pie	310
(Sara Lee Homestyle), 1/8 pie	340
(Sara Lee Reduced Fat), 1/6 pie	290
deep dish *(Mrs. Smith's Special Recipe),* 1/12 pie	330
Dutch *(Sara Lee* Homestyle), 1/8 pie	350
Dutch, crumb *(Mrs. Smith's),* 1/8 pie	350
banana cream *(Mrs. Smith's),* 1/4 pie	290
banana cream *(Pet-Ritz),* 1/3 pie	350
blueberry *(Sara Lee* Homestyle), 1/8 pie	360
Boston cream, see "Cake, frozen"	
cherry *(Mrs. Smith's),* 1/8 pie	310
cherry, deep dish *(Mrs. Smith's Special Recipe),* 1/12 pie	330
cherry-berry *(Mrs. Smith's Special Recipe),* 1/10 pie	360
chocolate, French silk *(Mrs. Smith's Restaurant Classics),* 1/9 pie	560
chocolate cream *(Mrs. Smith's),* 1/4 pie	330
chocolate cream *(Pet-Ritz),* 1/3 pie	340
coconut cream *(Mrs. Smith's),* 1/4 pie	340

coconut cream *(Pet-Ritz)*, ⅓ pie 350
coconut cream *(Sara Lee)*, ⅕ pie 480
cookies and cream *(Mrs. Smith's Restaurant Classics)*,
  ⅑ pie 390
fudge vanilla cream *(Pet-Ritz)*, ⅓ pie 350
key lime *(Mrs. Smith's Restaurant Classics)*, ⅑ pie 420
key lime cream *(Pet-Ritz)*, ⅓ pie 350
lemon cream *(Mrs. Smith's)*, ¼ pie 300
lemon cream *(Pet-Ritz)*, ⅓ pie 350
lemon meringue *(Mrs. Smith's)*, ⅕ pie 300
lemon meringue *(Sara Lee Homestyle)*, ⅙ pie 350
mince/mincemeat *(Sara Lee Homestyle)*, ⅛ pie 390
peach *(Sara Lee Homestyle)*, ⅛ pie 320
peach deep dish *(Mrs. Smith's Special Recipe)*, 1/12 pie . 300
peanut butter chocolate cream *(Pet-Ritz)*, ⅓ pie 370
peanut butter cream *(Mrs. Smith's)*, ¼ pie 360
peanut butter silk *(Mrs. Smith's Restaurant Classics)*,
  ⅑ pie 600
pecan *(Sara Lee Homestyle)*, ⅛ pie 520
pumpkin *(Mrs. Smith's Hearty)*, ⅛ pie 240
pumpkin *(Mrs. Smith's Special Recipe Homemade)*,
  1/10 pie 280
pumpkin *(Sara Lee Homestyle)*, ⅛ pie 260
pumpkin cream *(Pet-Ritz)*, ⅓ pie 350
pumpkin custard *(Mrs. Smith's)*, ⅛ pie 230
raspberry, red *(Sara Lee Homestyle)*, ⅛ pie 380
Pie, mix:
chocolate silk *(Jell-O No Bake)*, ⅙ pie 310
coconut cream *(Jell-O No Bake)*, ⅙ pie 330
Pie, snack, 1 pie, except as noted:
apple *(Entenmann's)*, 5-oz. pie 350
apple, blueberry, or peach *(Dolly Madison)*, 4.5-oz. pie . 480
blueberry *(Entenmann's)*, 5-oz. pie 420
cherry *(Dolly Madison)*, 4.5-oz. pie 470
cherry *(Entenmann's)*, 5-oz. pie 410
chocolate pudding *(Dolly Madison)*, 4.5-oz. pie 530
lemon *(Dolly Madison)*, 4.5-oz. pie 500
lemon *(Entenmann's)*, 5-oz. pie 430
peach *(Entenmann's)*, 5-oz. pie 380
pecan *(Dolly Madison)*, 3-oz. pie 360

Pie, snack *(cont.)*
pecan, fried *(Dolly Madison)*, 4.5-oz. pie 530
pineapple *(Dolly Madison)*, 4.5-oz. pie 460
pineapple *(Entenmann's)*, 5-oz. pie 400
Pie crust:
chocolate cookie *(Ready Crust)*, ⅛ crust 110
chocolate cookie *(Oreo)*, ⅙ crust 140
graham *(Honey Maid)*, ⅙ crust 140
graham *(Ready Crust 9″)*, ⅛ crust 110
graham *(Ready Crust 10″)* 1/10 crust 130
graham *(Ready Crust Low Fat 9″)*, ⅛ crust 100
graham, mini *(Ready Crust)*, .8-oz. crust 120
shortbread *(Ready Crust 9″)*, ⅛ crust 100
vanilla cookie *(Nilla)*, ⅙ crust 140
Pie crust, frozen or refrigerated:
(Oronoque 6″), ¼ crust 110
(Oronoque 9″), ⅛ crust 80
(Pet-Ritz 9″), ⅛ crust 80
(Pet-Ritz 9⅝″), ⅛ crust 120
(Pillsbury All Ready), ⅛ crust 120
deep dish *(Oronoque 9″)*, ⅛ crust 100
deep dish *(Oronoque 10″)*, ⅛ crust 120
deep dish *(Pet-Ritz 9″)*, ⅛ crust 90
graham *(Oronoque)*, ⅛ crust 110
vegetable shortening *(Pet-Ritz 9″)*, ⅛ crust 80
vegetable shortening deep dish *(Pet-Ritz)*, ⅛ crust 90
Pie crust mix *(Pillsbury)*, ⅛ of 9″ crust 100
Pie filling (see also "Pastry filling"), canned, ⅓ cup,
　　except as noted:
apple *(Comstock More Fruit)* 80
apple *(Lucky Leaf Lite)* 60
apple or apricot *(Lucky Leaf)* 90
berry, triple *(Crosse & Blackwell)* 120
blackberry *(Comstock)* 100
blueberry *(Lucky Leaf)* 100
blueberry *(Lucky Leaf Lite)* 60
cherry *(Lucky Leaf/Musselman's)* 100
cherry *(Lucky Leaf/Musselman's Lite)* 60
cherry, dark sweet *(Lucky Leaf/Musselman's)* 110
cherry blackberry *(Crosse & Blackwell)* 100

cherry cranberry *(Comstock)* 90
coconut creme *(Lucky Leaf)* 110
lemon or lemon cream *(Lucky Leaf/Musselman's)* 130
mincemeat *(Crosse & Blackwell)*, ¼ cup 180
mincemeat *(Comstock)* 170
mincemeat *(None Such)* 190
mincemeat, w/brandy and rum *(None Such)* 200
mincemeat, w/brandy and rum *(Crosse & Blackwell)*,
    ¼ cup 180
peach *(Lucky Leaf)* 80
pineapple *(Lucky Leaf/Musselman's)* 100
pumpkin, mix *(Libby's)* 90
raisin *(Lucky Leaf)* 100
strawberry *(Lucky Leaf/Musselman's)* 80
strawberry-rhubarb *(Lucky Leaf)* 90
Pie filling mix, see "Pudding mix"
Pie glaze, see "Glaze"
Pierogi, frozen or refrigerated:
potato cheese *(Old Fashioned Kitchen)*, 3 pieces, 1.4 oz. . 185
potato onion *(Giorgio)*, 3 pieces 230
potato onion *(Old Fashioned Kitchen)*, 3 pieces, 1.4 oz. . 182
Pigeon peas, ½ cup, except as noted:
fresh, boiled, drained 86
dried *(Goya)*, ¼ cup 140
dried, boiled 102
canned, dried *(El Jib)* 80
canned, dried, green *(Tupi)* 70
Pig's feet, pickled, cured, 1 oz. 58
Pignola nuts, see "Pine nuts"
Pike, meat only, 4 oz.:
northern, raw 100
northern, baked, broiled, or microwaved 128
walleye, raw 105
walleye, baked, broiled, or microwaved 135
Pili nuts, dried, shelled, 1 oz. 204
Pimiento, drained *(S&W)*, 2¼ oz. 20
Piña colada mixer, frozen* *(Bacardi)*, 8 fl. oz. 190
Pine nuts, dried:
pignolia *(Frieda's)*, ¼ cup, 1 oz. 150
pignolia *(Progresso)*, 1-oz. jar 170

Pine nuts *(cont.)*
pinyon, 1 oz. 161
pinyon, 10 kernels 6
Pineapple (see also "Pineapple, canned"):
fresh *(Frieda's* Sugar Loaf), ¾ cup, 3 oz. 30
fresh, diced, ½ cup 39
fresh, sliced *(Dole),* 2 slices 90
dried *(Sonoma),* 1.4 oz. 140
frozen, sweetened, chunks, ½ cup 104
Pineapple, candied *(Paradise/White Swan),* 1 oz. 90
Pineapple, canned, ½ cup, except as noted:
in juice, all varieties, except sliced *(Del Monte)* 70
in juice, crushed *(Dole)* 70
in juice, sliced *(Del Monte),* 2 slices, 4 oz. 60
in juice, sliced *(Dole),* 4 oz., 2 slices 60
in juice, tidbits *(Del Monte* Cup), 4 oz. 50
in juice, tidbits or chunks *(Dole)* 60
in light syrup, all varieties, except sliced *(Dole)* 80
in light syrup, sliced *(Dole),* 4 oz., 3½ slices 60
in light syrup, w/mandarin orange *(Dole)* 80
in heavy syrup, all varieties, except sliced *(Dole)* 90
in heavy syrup, crushed or chunks *(Del Monte)* 90
in heavy syrup, chunks, tidbits or crushed 100
in heavy syrup, sliced *(Del Monte),* 2 slices 90
in heavy syrup, sliced *(Dole),* 2 slices 90
in extra heavy syrup, crushed *(Dole)* 110
in extra heavy syrup, cubes *(Dole)* 200
Pineapple drink, mix*, 8 fl. oz., except as noted:
(Kool-Aid) 100
(Kool-Aid Presweetened) 60
Pineapple juice, 8 fl. oz.:
(Del Monte) 130
(Del Monte Not From Concentrate) 110
(Dole) 130
(Minute Maid) 130
Pineapple juice blend, 8 fl. oz.:
coconut *(R.W. Knudsen)* 130
guava *(Chiquita* Cocktail) 120
orange *(Tropicana)* 110
orange or orange-banana *(Dole)* 120

orange-strawberry *(Dole)* 130
Pineapple topping, 2 tbsp.:
(Kraft) 110
(Smucker's) 110
Pineapple-banana-orange smoothie *(Del Monte*
   Blenders), 6.25 fl. oz. 220
Pink beans, boiled, ½ cup 125
Pinto beans, ½ cup, except as noted:
dried *(Arrowhead Mills)*, ¼ cup 150
dried, boiled 117
canned *(Allens/East Texas Fair/Brown Beauty)* 110
canned *(Green Giant/Joan of Arc)* 110
canned *(Old El Paso)* 100
canned *(Progresso)* 110
canned, w/bacon *(Trappey's/Trappey's Jalapinto)* 120
Pinto beans, sprouted, boiled, drained, 4 oz. 25
Pistachio nut, shelled, except as noted:
dried, in shell *(River Queen)*, ½ cup, 1 oz. edible 170
dried *(Sonoma)*, ¼ cup 190
dry-roasted, 1 oz. 172
dry-roasted *(Planters)*, 1 oz. 160
Pita, see "Bread"
Pizza, frozen, 1 pie, except as noted:
bacon burger *(Totino's Pizza Party)*, ½ pie 380
Canadian bacon *(Jeno's Crisp 'n Tasty)* 440
Canadian bacon *(Tombstone* Original 12″), ¼ pie 360
Canadian bacon *(Totino's Pizza Party)*, ½ pie 330
cheese *(Amy's)*, 13 oz. 310
cheese *(Celeste* Large), ¼ pie 320
cheese *(Celeste* Large Premium), ¼ pie 350
cheese *(Celeste* for One) 420
cheese *(Jeno's Crisp 'n Tasty)* 460
cheese *(Tombstone For One* ½ Less Fat) 360
cheese *(Totino's* Family Size), ⅓ pie 370
cheese *(Totino's* Microwave for One) 240
cheese *(Totino's Pizza Party)*, ½ pie 320
cheese, extra *(Tombstone For One)* 540
cheese, extra *(Tombstone* Original 9″), ½ pie 420
cheese, extra *(Tombstone* Original 12″), ¼ pie 370
cheese, four *(Celeste* for One Original) 480

Pizza *(cont.)*

cheese, four *(Celeste* Rising Crust), ⅙ pie 340
cheese, four *(Tombstone Special Order* 12″), ⅕ pie 400
cheese, four, zesty *(Celeste* for One) 470
"cheese," nondairy *(Amy's* Soy Cheeze), 4.33 oz. 280
cheese, three, Italian style *(Tombstone* ThinCrust),
  ¼ pie 380
combination *(Jeno's Crisp 'n Tasty)* 520
comnination *(Totino's* Family Size), ⅓ pie 310
combination *(Totino's* Microwave for One) 310
combination *(Totino's Pizza Party)*, ½ pie 390
deluxe *(Celeste* Large), ¼ pie 350
deluxe *(Celeste* Large Premium), ¼ pie 390
deluxe *(Celeste* for One) 470
deluxe *(Tombstone* Original 9″), ⅓ pie 320
deluxe *(Tombstone* Original 12″), ⅕ pie 320
hamburger *(Jeno's Crisp 'n Tasty)* 500
hamburger *(Tombstone* Original 9″), ⅓ pie 310
hamburger *(Tombstone* Original 12″), ⅕ pie 320
hamburger *(Totino's Pizza Party)*, ½ pie 380
meat, four *(Tombstone Special Order* 9″), ⅓ pie 400
meat, four *(Tombstone Special Order* 12″), ⅙ pie 350
meat, four, combo, Italian *(Tombstone* ThinCrust),
  ¼ pie 410
meat, three *(Celeste* Rising Crust), ⅙ pie 390
meat, three *(Jeno's Crisp 'n Tasty)* 500
meat, three *(Totino's Pizza Party)*, ½ pie 360
Mexican style, supreme taco *(Tombstone* ThinCrust),
  ¼ pie 380
pepperoni *(Celeste* Large), ¼ pie 350
pepperoni *(Celeste* Large Premium), ¼ pie 390
pepperoni *(Celeste* for One) 470
pepperoni *(Celeste* Rising Crust), ⅙ pie 380
pepperoni *(Jeno's Crisp 'n Tasty)* 510
pepperoni *(Tombstone For One)* 580
pepperoni *(Tombstone* Original 12″), ⅕ pie 340
pepperoni *(Tombstone Special Order* 12″), ⅙ pie 360
pepperoni *(Totino's* Family Size), ⅓ pie 410
pepperoni *(Totino's* Microwave for One) 290
pepperoni *(Totino's Pizza Party)*, ½ pie 380

pepperoni, Italian style *(Tombstone* ThinCrust), ¼ pie . . . 420
pesto, w/tomatoes and broccoli *(Amy's),* 4.5 oz. 300
sausage *(Celeste* for One) 530
sausage *(Jeno's Crisp 'n Tasty)* 520
sausage *(Tombstone* Original 9″), ⅓ pie 310
sausage *(Tombstone* Original 12″), ⅕ pie 320
sausage *(Tombstone Special Order* 9″), ⅓ pie 390
sausage *(Totino's* Family Size), ⅓ pie 300
sausage *(Totino's* Microwave for One) 290
sausage *(Totino's Pizza Party),* ½ pie 380
sausage, w/double cheese *(Tombstone Double Top),*
  ⅙ pie 350
sausage, Italian *(Tombstone For One)* 560
sausage, Italian style *(Tombstone* ThinCrust), ¼ pie 400
sausage, three *(Tombstone Special Order* 12″), ⅙ pie . . . 340
sausage and mushroom *(Tombstone* Original 12″),
  ⅕ pie 320
sausage and mushroom *(Totino's Pizza Party),* ½ pie . . . 360
sausage and pepperoni *(Celeste* Large Premium), ¼ pie . 380
sausage and pepperoni *(Tombstone For One),* 1 pie 590
sausage and pepperoni *(Tombstone* Original 12″), ⅕ pie . 340
spinach *(Amy's),* 14 oz. 320
supreme *(Celeste* Rising Crust), ⅙ pie 380
supreme *(Celeste* Suprema Large), ⅕ pie 290
supreme *(Celeste* Suprema for One) 500
supreme *(Jeno's Crisp 'n Tasty)* 520
supreme *(Tombstone For One)* 570
supreme *(Tombstone For One* ½ Less Fat) 400
supreme *(Tombstone* Original 12″), ⅕ pie 330
supreme *(Tombstone Light),* ⅕ pie 270
supreme *(Totino's* Microwave for One) 300
supreme *(Totino's Pizza Party),* ½ pie 390
supreme, Italian style *(Tombstone* ThinCrust), ¼ pie 400
supreme, super *(Tombstone Special Order* 9″), ⅓ pie . . . 400
supreme, super *(Tombstone Special Order* 12″), ⅙ pie . . 350
vegetable *(Celeste* for One) 420
vegetable *(Tombstone For One* ½ Less Fat) 360
vegetable *(Tombstone Light),* ⅕ pie 240
vegetable, roasted *(Amy's),* 4 oz. 270

Pizza, French bread, frozen, 1 piece:

cheese *(Healthy Choice)*, 6 oz. 340
cheese *(Lean Cuisine)*, 6 oz. 320
cheese *(Stouffer's)*, 5.7 oz. 370
cheese, extra *(Stouffer's)*, 5.9 oz. 400
cheese, five *(Stouffer's)*, 5.1 oz. 420
deluxe *(Lean Cuisine)*, 6⅛ oz. 300
deluxe *(Stouffer's)*, 5.7 oz. 430
garlic, creamy *(Lean Cuisine)*, 6 oz. 310
meat, three *(Stouffer's)*, 6.25 oz. 460
pepperoni *(Healthy Choice)*, 6 oz. 340
pepperoni *(Lean Cuisine)*, 5¼ oz. 310
pepperoni *(Stouffer's)*, 5.6 oz. 430
pepperoni and mushroom *(Stouffer's)*, 6.1 oz. 440
sausage *(Healthy Choice)*, 6 oz. 320
sausage *(Stouffer's)*, 6 oz. 420
sausage and pepperoni *(Stouffer's)*, 6.25 oz. 470
sun-dried tomatoes *(Lean Cuisine)*, 6 oz. 340
supreme *(Healthy Choice)*, 6.35 oz. 330
vegetable *(Healthy Choice)*, 6 oz. 280
vegetable, grilled *(Stouffer's)*, 5.8 oz. 350
white *(Stouffer's)*, 5.1 oz. 460

Pizza burrito, see "Burrito"

Pizza crust:

refrigerated *(Pillsbury* All Ready), ⅕ crust 150
mix, dry *(Betty Crocker)*, ¼ crust 160
mix, dry *(Ragu Pizza Quick)*, ⅓ cup 130
mix, dry, deep pan *(Martha White)*, ⅕ pkg. 140
mix, dry, Italian herb *(Betty Crocker)*, ¼ crust 160

Pizza Hut, 1 slice of medium pie, except as noted:

Edge, medium:

   chicken/veggie 120
   meaty 150
   veggie 110
   works 140

Edge, large:

   chicken/veggie 160
   meaty 200
   veggie 140
   works 180

hand-tossed:
    beef or cheese 280
    chicken supreme 240
    ham 230
    Meat Lover's, super supreme, or pork topping 290
    pepperoni 260
    Pepperoni Lover's 320
    sausage, Italian 300
    supreme 250
    Veggie Lover's 240
pan pizza:
    beef 310
    cheese 300
    chicken supreme or pepperoni 280
    ham 250
    Meat Lover's 360
    Pepperoni Lover's or Italian sausage 350
    pork topping or supreme 300
    super supreme 340
    Veggie Lover's 240
Pizzeria Stuffed Crust:
    beef or pepperoni 410
    cheese or ham 380
    chicken supreme 390
    Meat Lover's 500
    Pepperoni Lover's 480
    pork topping 420
    sausage, Italian 430
    super supreme 470
    supreme 440
    Veggie Lover's 390
Sicilian:
    beef 320
    cheese or pepperoni 290
    chicken supreme 270
    ham 260
    Meat Lover's 350
    Pepperoni Lover's or Italian sausage 330
    super supreme or pork topping 320
    supreme 310

Pizza Hut, Sicilian *(cont.)*
   Veggie Lover's 270
Thin 'N Crispy:
   beef 240
   cheese 210
   chicken supreme 220
   ham 190
   Meat Lover's 310
   pepperoni 220
   Pepperoni Lovers or pork topping 270
   sausage, Italian 300
   super supreme 280
   supreme 250
   Veggie Lover's 170
starters/sides:
   Buffalo wings, hot, 4 pieces 210
   Buffalo wings, mild, 5 pieces 200
   garlic bread, 1 slice 150
   bread stick, 1 piece 130
   bread stick dipping sauce 30
Pizza pepper *(Lawry's)*, ¼ tsp. 0
Pizza pocket, frozen, 4.5-oz. piece:
(Ken & Robert's Veggie Pockets) 270
cheese *(Amy's)* 290
pepperoni *(Croissant Pockets)* 360
pepperoni *(Deli Stuffs)* 350
pepperoni *(Hot Pockets)* 350
pepperoni deluxe *(Lean Pockets)* 270
pepperoni and sausage *(Hot Pockets)* 330
sausage *(Hot Pockets)* 340
supreme *(Croissant Pockets)* 390
vegetarian *(Amy's)* 240
Pizza sauce, ¼ cup:
(Muir Glen) 40
(Prince Traditional Arabic), ¼ cup 20
(Progresso) 20
(Ragú Pizza Quick 100% Natural) 30
(Ragú Pizza Quick Traditional) 40
garlic and basil *(Ragú Pizza Quick)* 40
mushroom, chunky *(Ragú Pizza Quick)* 40

pepperoni flavored *(Ragú Pizza Quick)* 60
tomato, chunky *(Ragú Pizza Quick)* 50
Pizza seasoning *(Tone's Presti's)*, ¾ tsp. 10
Pizza stuffed sandwich, see "Pizza pocket"
Plantain, raw *(Frieda's)*, 3 oz. 100
Plum:
fresh, Japanese or hybrid, 2⅛″ fruit 36
fresh, sliced, ½ cup 46
canned, in juice, ½ cup 73
canned, in juice, 3 plums and 2 tbsp. liquid 55
canned, in light syrup, ½ cup 79
canned, in light syrup, 3 plums and 2¾ tbsp. liquid 83
canned, heavy syrup, ½ cup 115
Plum sauce:
(Ka•Me), 2 tbsp. 70
dipping *(Trader Vic's)*, 2 tbsp. 70
Poi, ½ cup 134
Polenta (see also "Cornmeal"), dry *(Contadina)*, 3 tbsp. . 110
Polenta, prepared:
plain *(Frieda's)*, 4 oz. 100
plain *(San Gennaro)*, 2 slices, ½″ 70
basil and garlic *(San Gennaro)*, 2 slices, ½″ 71
sundried tomato *(San Gennaro)*, 2 slices, ½″ 74
Polenta dishes, mix, dry, 1.8-oz. cup, except as noted:
(Fantastic Foods International Fantastica), ⅜ cup 260
cheese, three *(Fantastic Foods* Cup) 210
Mediterranean *(Fantastic Foods* Cup) 200
Mexicana, spicy *(Fantastic Foods* Cup) 210
Santa Fe *(Fantastic Foods* Cup) 220
Polenta entree, ½ pkg.:
mushroom and onion, w/chicken sausage sauce *(San
Gennaro)* 130
green chili and cilantro, w/black bean sauce *(San
Gennaro)* 140
spinach and cheese, w/marinara sauce *(San Gennaro)* . . . 120
Polenta mix *(Fantastica)*, 1 cup* 260
Polish sausage (see also "Kielbasa"):
(Ball Park), 3-oz. link 240
beef *(Hebrew National)*, 3-oz. link 240
hot *(Ball Park)*, 3-oz. link 240

Pollock, meat only, 4 oz.:

Atlantic, raw 104
Atlantic, baked, broiled, or microwaved 134
walleye, raw 91
walleye, baked, broiled, or microwaved 128
Pomegranate, 9.7-oz. fruit 104
Pomegranate juice *(R.W. Knudsen),* 8 fl. oz. 150
Pomegranate syrup, see "Grenadine"
Pompano, Florida, meat only:

raw, 4 oz. 186
baked, broiled, or microwaved, 4 oz. 239
Popcorn:

(Jolly Time Microwave Natural), 2 tbsp., 4 cups popped . 150
(Jolly Time Microwave Natural Light), 2 tbsp., 4 cups
   popped 120
(Pop•Secret Homestyle/Natural), 3 tbsp. 170
(Pop•Secret Natural Light), 3 tbsp. 140
(Pop•Secret Natural 99% Fat Free), 3 tbsp. 120
butter/butter flavor:

   (America's Best), 2 tbsp., 5 cups popped 90
   (Jolly Time Blast O Butter), 2 tbsp., 3.5 cups
      popped 150
   (Jolly Time Blast O Butter Light), 2 tbsp., 4 cups
      popped 130
   (Jolly Time Butter 'Licious), 2 tbsp., 4 cups popped . 140
   (Jolly Time Butter 'Licious Light), 2 tbsp., 4 cups
      popped 120
   (Pop•Secret), 3 tbsp. 170
   (Pop•Secret 99% Fat Free), 3 tbsp. 120
   (Pop•Secret Snack Size), 1/4 cup 230
   (Pop•Secret Land O Lakes/Movie Theater), 3 tbsp. . . . 180
   (Pop•Secret Jumbo Pop), 3 tbsp. 170
   light *(Pop•Secret),* 3 tbsp. 140
   light *(Pop•Secret Movie Theater),* 3 tbsp. 140
cheddar *(Jolly Time* Microwave), 2 tbsp., 3 cups
   popped 160
cheddar *(Pop•Secret),* 3 tbsp. 180
cheddar *(Pop•Secret),* 5 cups popped 150
Popcorn, popped:

(Frieda's), 2 cups 120

(Northern Lites 50% Less Fat), 4 cups 130
(Wise Baby White Lowfat) 2½ cups 140
butter/butter flavor:
   (Chester's), 3 cups 160
   (Chester's Microwave), 5 cups 200
   (Old Dutch Gourmet White), 2¾ cups 160
   (Smartfood), 3 cups 150
   (Wise), 1-oz. bag 150
   (Wise Lite), 4 cups 140
caramel *(Chester's),* ¾ cup 130
caramel *(Smart Snackers),* 9 oz. 100
caramel *(Wise* Choice Fat Free), ¾ cup 110
caramel w/peanuts *(Cracker Jacks),* ½ cup 120
caramel w/peanuts *(Cracker Jacks* Fat Free), ¾ cup 110
caramel w/peanuts *(Moore's),* ¾ cup 110
cheese flavored *(Moore's),* 2 cups 160
cheese flavored, cheddar *(Wise* Buttery), 2 cups 160
cheese flavored, hot *(Wise/Moore's),* 2 cups 150
cheddar, white *(Chester's),* 3 cups 190
cheddar, white *(Old Dutch* Premium), 2⅓ cups 160
cheddar, white *(Smartfood),* 2 cups 190
cheddar, white *(Wise),* 2 cups 160
cheddar, yellow *(Old Dutch),* 2½ cups 160
toffee, butter *(Cracker Jacks* Fat Free), ¾ cup 110
toffee, butter *(Wise* Fat Free), ¾ cup 110
toffee crunch *(Smartfood* Lowfat), ¾ cup 110
Poppy seed, 1 tsp. 15
Poppy seed filling, see "Pastry filling"
Porgy, see "Scup"
Pork (see also "Ham"), meat only, 4 oz., except as
  noted:
loin, whole, roasted, lean w/fat 362
loin, whole, roasted, lean only 272
loin, blade, broiled, lean w/fat 446
loin, blade, broiled, lean only 340
loin, blade, roasted, lean w/fat 413
loin, blade, roasted, lean only 316
loin, center:
   broiled, lean w/fat 358

Pork, loin, center *(cont.)*

broiled, lean w/fat, 3.1 oz. (3.7 oz. raw chop w/ bone)	275
broiled, lean only	262
broiled, lean only, 2.5 oz. (3.7 oz. raw chop w/bone and fat)	166
roasted, lean w/fat	346
roasted, lean only	272
loin, center rib:	
broiled, lean w/fat	389
broiled, lean only	293
roasted, lean w/fat	361
roasted, lean only	278
loin, top, broiled, lean w/fat	408
loin, top, broiled, lean only	293
loin, top, roasted, lean only	278
shoulder, whole, roasted, lean w/fat	370
shoulder, whole, roasted, lean only	277
shoulder, arm (picnic), roasted, lean w/fat	375
shoulder, arm (picnic), roasted, lean only	259
shoulder, arm (picnic), roasted, lean only, diced, 1 cup	319
shoulder, Boston blade, braised, lean w/fat	421
shoulder, Boston blade, braised, lean only	333
shoulder, Boston blade, broiled, lean w/fat	397
shoulder, Boston blade, broiled, lean only	311
shoulder, Boston blade, roasted, lean only	290
sirloin:	
broiled, lean w/fat	375
broiled, lean w/fat, 3 oz. (3.7 oz. raw chop w/bone)	278
broiled, lean only	276
broiled, lean only, 2.4 oz. (3.7 oz. raw chop w/bone and fat)	165
roasted, lean w/fat	330
roasted, lean only	268
spareribs, lean w/fat, braised, 6.3 oz. (1 lb. raw w/ bone)	703
tenderloin, lean only, roasted	188
Pork, cured (see also "Ham"), 4 oz.:	
arm (picnic), roasted, lean w/fat	318
arm (picnic), roasted, lean only	193

blade roll, lean w/fat, roasted 325
Pork, refrigerated:
barbecue sauce, w/shredded pork *(Lloyd's)*, ¼ cup 90
spareribs *(Lloyd's)*, 3 ribs w/sauce, 5 oz. 380
Pork batter, frying *(House of Tsang)*, 4 tbsp. 140
Pork belly, raw, 1 oz. 147
Pork dinner, frozen, 1 pkg.:
chop, country fried *(Marie Callender's)*, 15 oz. 550
riblet, boneless *(Banquet Extra Helping)*, 15.25 oz. 720
Pork entree, frozen, 1 pkg.:
cutlet *(Banquet Meal)*, 10.25 oz. 420
cutlet, breaded *(Stouffer's Homestyle)*, 10 oz. 420
honey roasted *(Lean Cuisine Cafe Classics)*, 9½ oz. 250
patty, grilled, glazed *(Healthy Choice)*, 9.6 oz. 300
and roasted potatoes *(Stouffer's Hearty Portions)*, 15⅜
   oz. 540
riblet, boneless *(Banquet Meal)*, 10 oz. 400
Pork gravy, canned *(Franco-American Golden)*, ¼ cup . . . 45
Pork lunch meat, seasoned *(Boar's Head)*, 2 oz. 80
Pork rind snack, ½ oz.:
(Baken-ets/Baken-ets Cracklins) 80
hot and spicy *(Baken-ets)* 70
hot and spicy *(Baken-ets Cracklins)* 80
Pork seasoning mix:
(Durkee/French's Roasting Bag), ⅙ pkg. 25
(Shake'n Bake Original Recipe), ⅛ pkg. 40
barbecue glaze *(Shake'n Bake)*, ⅛ pkg. 35
extra crispy *(Oven Fry)*, ⅛ pkg. 60
hot and spicy *(Shake'n Bake)*, ⅛ pkg. 45
sparerib *(Durkee Roasting Bag)*, ⅐ pkg. 25
Posole, see "Corn, dried"
Pot pie, see specific entrée listings
Pot roast, see "Beef dinner" and "Beef entree"
Potato:
raw, all varieties *(Frieda's)*, ½ cup, 3 oz. 70
baked, in skin, 4¾″ × 2⅓″ 220
boiled in skin, baby *(Frieda's)*, 4 oz. 86
boiled in skin, peeled, 2½″ potato 119
boiled w/out skin, 2½″ potato 116
boiled, w/out skin, ½ cup 67

Potato *(cont.)*
microwaved in skin, 4¾″ × 2⅓″ potato 212
mashed, w/whole milk, and butter or margarine, ½ cup . 111
Potato, canned:
whole *(Seneca/Seneca No Salt)*, ⅔ cup 80
whole, new *(Del Monte)*, 2 medium w/liquid 60
sliced *(Del Monte)*, ⅔ cup 60
Potato, frozen (see also "Potato dishes, frozen"), 3 oz.,
   except as noted:
au gratin *(Cascadian Farm)*, ⅔ cup 110
fried *(Cascadian Farm Oven French Fries)* 130
fried *(Ore-Ida Deep Fries/Deep Fries Crinkle Cut)* 160
fried *(Ore-Ida Shoestrings)* 150
fried *(Ore-Ida Steak Fries)* 110
fried *(Ore-Ida Crispers!)* 220
fried *(Ore-Ida Golden Crinkles)* 140
fried *(Ore-Ida Golden Pixie Crinkles)* 130
fried *(Ore-Ida Waffle Fries)* 150
fried, cottage fries *(Ore-Ida)* 130
hash browns *(Cascadian Farm)*, 1 cup 70
hash browns *(Ore-Ida Golden Patties)*, 1 piece 160
hash browns, w/cheddar *(Ore-Ida Cheddar Browns)*,
   1 piece 80
has browns, shredded *(Ore-Ida)*, 1 piece 70
O'Brien *(Ore-Ida)*, ¾ cup 60
w/peppers and onions *(Cascadian Farm Country Style)*,
   ¾ cup 80
puffs *(Cascadian Farm Spud Puppies)* 150
puffs *(Tater Tots)* 160
Potato, mix, see "Potato dishes, mix"
Potato, refrigerated, mashed *(Diner's Choice)*, ⅔ cup . . 110
Potato, stuffed, see "Potato dishes"
Potato, sweet, see "Sweet potato"
Potato chips and crisps, 1 oz., except as noted:
(Herr's Ripples) 140
(Lay's) 150
(Lay's Adobadas) 170
(Lay's Baked) 110
(Lay's Wavy) 160
(Lay's/Ruffles WOW Original) 75

(Munchos)	150
(Ruffles)	150
(Ruffles Baked)	110
(Ruffles Reduced Fat)	130
(Sun Chips)	140
(Wise)	150
barbecue *(Lay's KC Masterpiece*/Red Hot Pepper Grill)	150
barbecue *(Lay's KC Masterpiece* Baked)	120
barbecue *(Munchos)*	160
barbecue *(Wise)*	160
barbecue, mesquite *(Kettle* Chips)	130
barbecue, mesquite *(Lay's WOW)*	75
barbecue, mesquite *(Ruffles KC Masterpiece)*	150
barbecue, mesquite *(Wise Krunchers!)*	140
cheddar *(Andy Capp Cheddar Fries)*	140
cheddar *(Lay's* Deli Style)	150
cheddar/sour cream *(Ruffles)*	160
cheddar/sour cream *(Ruffles* Baked)	120
cheddar/sour cream *(Wise)*	160
cheese, au gratin *(Lay's* Wavy)	150
chili *(Lay's* Deli Style)	150
Dijon, golden *(Ruffles)*	150
dill *(Wise)*	150
hot *(Andy Capp Hot Fries)*	140
hot *(Lay's* Flamin')	150
hot *(Wise)*	150
jalapeño *(Wise Krunchers!)*	140
jalapeño, cheddar *(Kettle* Chips)	130
jalapeño jack *(Wise)*	150
onion, French *(Ruffles)*	150
onion, French *(Sun Chips)*	140
onion and garlic *(Lay's)*	150
onion and garlic *(Wise)*	150
ranch *(Lay's Hidden Valley* Wavy)	160
ranch *(Ruffles)*	150
salsa *(Andy Capp Salsa Fries)*	130
salt and vinegar *(Lay's)*	150
salt and vinegar *(Wise)*	150
sour cream/onion *(Lay's)*	160

Potato chips and crisps *(cont.)*
sour cream/onion *(Lay's Baked)* 120
sour cream/onion *(Ruffles Reduced Fat)* 130
sour cream/onion *(Wise)* 150
sticks *(French's)*, ¾-oz. bag 120
sticks, hot *(Chester's Fries Flamin')* 140
sweet, spicy *(Wise Mambo Mania)* 160
Potato dishes, frozen, 1 pkg., except as noted:
au gratin *(Stouffer's Side Dish)*, ½ cup 150
au gratin, ham and broccoli *(Banquet Family)*, ⅔ cup . . . 210
casserole, garden *(Healthy Choice)*, 9.25 oz. 210
cheddar *(Lean Cuisine Deluxe)*, 10⅜ oz. 270
cheddar, broccoli *(Healthy Choice)*, 10.5 oz. 330
roasted, w/broccoli and cheddar sauce *(Lean Cuisine)*,
    10¼ oz. 260
scalloped *(Stouffer's Entree/Side Dish)*, ½ cup 140
scalloped, w/smoked turkey ham *(Lean Cuisine
    American Favorites)*, 10 oz. 250
wedges, cheese, broccoli, bacon *(Marie Callender's)*,
    13 oz. 420
wedges, w/Swiss, chicken *(Marie Callender's)*, 13 oz. . . . 390
wedges, w/Swiss, ham, and broccoli *(Marie
    Callender's)*, 13 oz. 380
Potato dishes, mix, ½ cup*, except as noted:
(Betty Crocker Potato Shakers Original), ⅔ cup* 140
au gratin *(Betty Crocker)* 150
au gratin *(Hungry Jack)* 150
chicken/vegetable *(Betty Crocker)*, ⅔ cup* 140
broccoli au gratin *(Betty Crocker)* 140
cheddar *(Betty Crocker)* 120
cheddar/bacon *(Betty Crocker)* 150
cheddar/bacon *(Hungry Jack)* 150
cheddar/bacon, twice baked *(Betty Crocker)*, ⅔ cup* . . . 210
cheddar/sour cream *(Betty Crocker)* 130
cheese, three *(Betty Crocker)* 150
hash browns *(Betty Crocker)* 190
julienne *(Betty Crocker)* 150
mashed *(Betty Crocker Potato Buds)*, ⅔ cup* 160
mashed *(Hungry Jack Flakes)* 160
mashed *(Hungry Jack Idaho Flakes)* 150

mashed *(Hungry Jack* Idaho Granules) 160
mashed, butter flavor, garlic, or parsley *(Hungry Jack)* . . 150
mashed, butter and herb *(Betty Crocker)* 160
mashed, cheese, 4, or chicken and herb *(Betty Crocker)* . 150
mashed, sour cream/chive *(Betty Crocker)* 150
mashed, stuffed, 1 pkg., except as noted:
  broccoli cheddar *(Fantastic Foods),* ¼ cup 100
  broccoli cheddar *(Fantastic Foods* Cup) 190
  butter, creamery *(Fantastic Foods* Cup) 200
  cheddar *(Fantastic Foods),* ¼ cup 100
  cheddar *(Fantastic Foods* Cup) 180
  garlic and herbs *(Fantastic Foods),* ¼ cup 100
  garlic and herbs *(Fantastic Foods* Cup) 180
  jalapeño jack cheese *(Fantastic Foods* Cup) 200
  sour cream and chive *(Fantastic Foods),* ¼ cup 100
  sour cream/chives *(Fantastic Foods* Cup) 180
scalloped *(Betty Crocker* 8.25 oz.) 150
scalloped, cheesy *(Betty Crocker)* 140
scalloped, cheesy or creamy *(Hungry Jack)* 150
scalloped or ranch *(Betty Crocker)* 160
sour cream/chive *(Betty Crocker)* 160
sour cream/chive *(Hungry Jack)* 160
Potato entree, frozen, see "Potato dishes"
Potato entree, packaged, w/curried garbanzos, rice
  (Tamarind Tree Alu Chole), 1 pkg. 350
Potato pancake mix:
(Hungry Jack), 2 tbsp. 70
(Hungry Jack), 3 cakes*, 3″ 90
(Manischewitz), 3 tbsp., 3 cakes* 80
latke *(Manischewitz),* 2 tbsp, 3 latkes* 80
Potato seasoning:
cheddar, crispy *(Shake'n Bake),* ⅙ pkt. 30
cheddar, savory *(Lipton Recipe Secrets),* 1 tbsp. 60
garlic herb *(Lipton Recipe Secrets),* 1 tbsp. 50
herb and garlic *(Shake'n Bake),* ⅙ pkt. 20
onion, California *(Lipton Recipe Secrets)* 60
Potato sticks, see "Potato chips and crisps"
Potato-cheddar pocket, frozen *(Ken & Robert's Veggie
  Pockets),* 1 piece 260

Poultry, see specific listings
Poultry seasoning, 1 tsp. 5
Pout, ocean, meat only:
raw, 4 oz. 90
baked, broiled, or microwaved, 4 oz. 116
Preserves, see "Jam and preserves"
Pretzels:
(Mister Salty Mini), 1 oz. 110
bagel shaped *(Manischewitz),* 4 pieces, 1 oz. 110
beer *(Quinlan),* 2 pieces, 1 oz. 110
cheese *(Handi-Snacks),* 1.1-oz. piece 110
cheese *(Sargento MooTown Snackers),* .9-oz. piece 90
Dutch *(Mister Salty),* 2 pieces, 1.1 oz. 120
hard, plain, 1 oz. 108
mini *(Quinlan Fat Free/No Salt Added),* 1 oz. 100
mustard, honey *(Rold Gold),* 1 oz. 110
nuggets *(Quinlan),* 17 pieces, 1 oz. 110
oat bran nuggets *(Smart Snackers),* 1½ oz. 170
rods *(Quinlan Rods/Logs),* 3 pieces, 1 oz. 110
rods *(Rold Gold),* 1 oz. 110
soft *(Superpretzel),* 2.3-oz. piece 170
soft, cheese *(Superpretzel Softstix),* 2 pieces, 1.8 oz. . . . 140
sourdough *(Quinlan Low Fat),* 1 piece, .9 oz. 90
sourdough, hard *(Rold Gold* Nuggets), 1 oz. 110
sourdough, nuggets *(Quinlan* San Francisco), 1 oz. 110
sticks *(Bachman Stix),* 1 oz. 100
sticks *(Quinlan),* 1 oz. 110
sticks *(Quinlan Fat Free),* 1 oz. 100
sticks *(Rold Gold Fat Free),* 1 oz. 110
thins *(Quinlan Fat Free),* 1 oz. 100
thins *(Quinlan/Quinlan Party),* 1 oz. 110
thins *(Rold Gold Crispy's/Fat Free),* 1 oz. 110
twists, *(Mister Salty),* 1 oz. 110
twists, tiny *(Rold Gold Fat Free),* 1 oz. 100
Prickly pear, 1 medium, 4.8 oz. 42
Profiterole, frozen *(Manzoni),* 3.5 oz. 320
Prosciutto *(Boar's Head),* 1 oz. 60
Prune:
canned, in heavy syrup, ½ cup 123

canned, stewed *(S&W)*, 8 pieces, 4.9 oz. 210
dried, w/pits, ½ cup 193
dried, pitted, 10 prunes 201
dried, stewed, w/pits, unsweetened, ½ cup 113
Prune juice *(R.W. Knudsen)*, 8 fl. oz. 170
Pudding, 4 oz., except as noted:
banana *(Imagine)*, 3.7-oz. cup 140
banana *(Jell-O)* 170
banana *(Kozy Shack)* 130
butterscotch *(Imagine)*, 3.7-oz. cup 140
chocolate *(Imagine)*, 3.7-oz. cup 160
chocolate *(Jell-O)* 160
chocolate *(Jell-O Free)* 100
chocolate *(Kozy Shack)* 140
chocolate, light *(Kozy Shack)* 110
chocolate-caramel or vanilla swirl *(Jell-O)* 160
chocolate-vanilla swirl *(Jell-O Free)* 100
flan/creme caramel *(Kozy Shack)* 150
lemon *(Imagine)*, 3.7-oz. cup 150
rice, see "Rice pudding"
tapioca *(Jell-O)* 140
tapioca *(Kozy Shack)* 140
vanilla *(Jell-O)* 160
vanilla *(Jell-O Free)* 100
vanilla *(Kozy Shack)* 130
vanilla-chocolate swirl *(Jell-O)* 160
vanilla-chocolate swirl *(Jell-O Free)* 100
Pudding, mix, ½ cup*, except as noted:
banana *(Jell-O Sugar/Fat Free)* 70
banana cream *(Jell-O)* 140
banana cream *(Jell-O Instant)* 150
butter pecan *(Jell-O Instant)* 160
butterscotch *(Jell-O)* 160
butterscotch *(Jell-O Instant)* 150
butterscotch *(Jell-O Sugar/Fat Free)* 70
chocolate *(Jell-O)* 150
chocolate *(Jell-O Instant)* 160
chocolate *(Jell-O Sugar Free)* 90
chocolate *(Jell-O Sugar/Fat Free)* 80

Pudding, mix *(cont.)*
chocolate, milk or fudge *(Jell-O)* 150
chocolate milk or fudge *(Jell-O* Instant) 160
chocolate fudge *(Jell-O* Sugar/Fat Free) 80
chocolate mousse, see "Mousse mix"
coconut cream *(Jell-O)* 150
coconut cream *(Jell-O* Instant) 160
custard *(Jello-O Americana)* 140
flan *(Alsa* Creme Caramel), 1⅓ tbsp. mix, 1 tbsp.
  caramel 110
flan *(Jell-O)* 140
lemon *(Jell-O)* 140
lemon *(Jell-O* Instant) 150
pistachio *(Jell-O* Instant) 160
pistachio *(Jell-O* Sugar/Fat Free) 70
rice, see "Rice pudding mix"
tapioca *(Jell-O Americana)* 140
vanilla *(Jell-O)* 140
vanilla *(Jell-O* Instant) 150
vanilla *(Jell-O* Sugar Free) 80
vanilla *(Jell-O* Sugar/Fat Free) 70
vanilla, French *(Jell-O* Instant) 150
Pudding, plum *(Crosse & Blackwell)*, ⅓ pkg. 410
Pudding bar, frozen, all flavors *(Eskimo Pie)*, 1 bar 90
Pummelo, sections, ½ cup 36
Pumpkin, ½ cup:
fresh, pulp, raw, 1″ cubes 15
fresh, boiled, drained, mashed 24
canned *(Libby's* Solid Pack) 40
pie mix, see "Pie filling"
Pumpkin butter *(Smucker's)*, 1 tbsp. 45
Pumpkin pie spice, 1 tsp. 6
Pumpkin seeds:
roasted, in shell, 1 oz. or 85 seeds 127
roasted, shelled, 1 oz. 148
dried, shelled, 1 oz. or 142 kernels 154
Punch, see "Fruit punch" and specific fruit listings
Quail, raw:
meat w/skin, 1 quail, 3.8 oz. (4.3 oz. w/bone) 210
meat only, 1 quail, 3.2 oz. (4.3 oz. w/bone and skin) 123

breast meat only, 1 breast, 2 oz. 69
Quesadilla dip, w/chicken *(Tostitos),* 4 tbsp. 50
Quince, 1 medium, 5.3 oz. 53
Quinoa, dry *(Frieda's),* 1/3 cup 170
Quinoa seeds *(Arrowhead Mills),* 1/4 cup 140

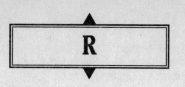

FOOD AND MEASURE   **CALORIES**

Rabbit, meat only:
domesticated, roasted, 4 oz. 223
domesticated, stewed, 4 oz. 234
wild, stewed, 4 oz. 196
Radiatore pasta dishes, mix, dry:
spicy tomato sauce *(DeBoles)*, 2 oz. 240
w/sun-dried tomato-basil sauce *(Annie's)*, ²/₃ cup 260
Radicchio, fresh *(Frieda's)*, 2 cups, 3 oz. 20
Radish, 10 medium, ³/₄"–1" 7
Radish, black *(Frieda's)*, ³/₄ cup, 3 oz. 15
Radish, Chinese *(Frieda's* Lo Bok)*, ²/₃ cup, 3 oz. 25
Radish, Oriental:
(Frieda's Daikon)*, ²/₃ cup, 3 oz. 15
raw, sliced, ¹/₂ cup 8
boiled, drained, sliced, ¹/₂ cup 13
Radish, white-icicle, 1 medium, .6 oz. 2
Raisin, ¹/₄ cup:
golden seedless, not packed 110
seedless, not packed 109
chocolate or yogurt coated, see "Candy"
Ranch dip, 2 tbsp:
(Heluva Good)* 60
(Heluva Good Fat Free)* 25
(Kraft) 60
(Ruffles) 70
(Ruffles Lowfat)* 40
Ranch dip mix, 2 tbsp.*:
(Hidden Valley Fiesta)* 70
(Hidden Valley Original)* 70
(Hidden Valley Original Reduced Calorie)* 40
Rapini, see "Broccoli rabe"
Raspberry, red:
fresh, ¹/₂ cup 31
frozen *(Cascadian Farm)*, 1 cup 60

frozen, sweetened, ½ cup 129
Raspberry drink, lemon *(Dole* Splash), 8 fl. oz. 120
Raspberry juice *(Dole* Country), 8 fl. oz. 140
Raspberry syrup, red *(Smucker's),* ¼ cup 210
Raspberry-tamarind dipping sauce *(Helen's Tropical*
   Exotics), 2 tbsp. 50
Ravioli, frozen or refrigerated, 1 cup, except as noted:
cheese, four *(Contadina)* 290
cheese, four *(Contadina* Light) 230
cheese, Italian herb *(Di Giorno)* 350
cheese, w/Italian sausage *(Di Giorno),* ¾ cup 340
cheese and garlic *(Di Giorno Light Varieties)* 270
beef and garlic *(Contadina)* 330
chicken, smoked *(Contadina)* 240
chicken and herb *(Contadina),* 1¼ cups 370
gorgonzola *(Contadina),* 1¼ cups 360
tomato and cheese *(Di Giorno Light Varieties)* 280
vegetable, garden *(Contadina)* 250
Ravioli entree, canned, 1 cup, except as noted:
beef *(Progresso)* 260
beef, in meat sauce *(Franco-American Superiore)* 280
beef, w/pasta in tomato and cheese *(Franco-American)* . . 230
cheese *(Progresso)* 220
Ravioli entree, frozen, cheese, 1 pkg.:
(Lean Cuisine), 8½ oz. 270
(Stouffer's), 10⅝ oz. 380
parmigiana *(Healthy Choice),* 9 oz. 260
ricotta, w/sauce *(Amy's),* 9.5 oz. 340
Red beans (see also "Kidney beans"), canned, ½ cup:
(Allens) 160
(Green Giant/Joan of Arc) 100
Red snapper, see "Snapper"
Redfish, see "Ocean perch"
Refried beans, canned, ½ cup:
(Allens) 150
(Old El Paso/Old El Paso Fat Free) 100
(Ortega) 130
black beans *(Old El Paso)* 110
w/cheese *(Old El Paso)* 130
w/green chilies, spicy, or vegetarian *(Old El Paso)* 100

w/sausage *(Old El Paso)* 200
Refried beans, mix, dry, instant *(Fantastic Foods)*,
⅓ cup 160
Relish, see "Pickle-relish" and specific listings
Remoulade sauce *(Zararain's)*, ¼ cup 80
Rennet *(Junket)*, 1 tablet 1
Rhubarb:
fresh *(Frieda's)*, ⅔ cup, 3 oz. 20
fresh, diced, ½ cup 13
frozen, cooked, sweetened, ½ cup 139
Rice (see also "Wild rice"), dry, ¼ cup, except as
noted:
Arborio *(Fantastic Foods)* 210
basmati, brown *(Arrowhead Mills)* 150
basmati, brown *(Fantastic Foods)* 170
basmati, white *(Fantastic Foods)* 180
basmati, white, long grain *(Arrowhead Mills)* 150
brown *(Carolina/Mahatma/River)* 150
brown *(Success)*, ½ cup 150
brown, long grain *(Arrowhead Mills)* 150
brown, short grain *(Arrowhead Mills)* 170
brown, whole grain *(Minute* Instant), ½ cup 170
jasmine *(Fantastic Foods)* 170
white, long grain *(Carolina)* 150
white, long grain *(River/Water Maid)* 160
white, long grain *(Success)*, ½ cup 190
white, long grain, instant *(Carolina)* 160
white, long grain, instant *(Minute)*, ½ cup 170
white, long grain, instant *(Minute* Boil-in-Bag), ½ cup . . 190
Rice bran, crude, 1 cup 262
Rice cake, 1 cake:
all varieties *(Lundberg)* 60
all varieties, bars *(Health Valley* Crisp Fat Free) 110
cheese, cheddar *(Crispy Cakes)* 35
cheese, cheddar or nacho corn *(Quaker)* 40
cinnamon crunch *(Quaker)* 50
multigrain *(Mother's)* 35
pizza or ranch *(Crispy Cakes)* 30
vegetable, garden *(Crispy Cakes)* 35
wheat *(Quaker)* 35

Rice dishes, canned, Spanish *(Old El Paso),* 1 cup . . . 130
Rice dishes, frozen (see also "Rice entree, frozen"),
   1 pkg.:
and broccoli *(Green Giant)* 320
w/vegetables *(Green Giant* Medley) 240
w/vegetables:
   Caribbean *(Cascadian Farm Veggie Bowl),* 9 oz. . . . 280
   fiesta *(Cascadian Farm Veggie Bowl),* 9 oz. 340
   Madras curry *(Cascadian Farm Veggie Bowl),* 9 oz. . . . 270
   pilaf *(Green Giant)* 230
   Szechuan *(Cascadian Farm Veggie Bowl),* 9 oz. 210
   teriyaki *(Cascadian Farm Veggie Bowl),* 9 oz. 270
   white and wild *(Green Giant)* 250
Rice dishes, mix, 2 oz. dry, except as noted:
Alfredo broccoli *(Lipton* Rice & Sauce), 1 cup* 320
and beans:
   black *(Mahatma)* 200
   black, Jamaican *(Fantastic Foods Healthy*
     Complements), 1/3 cup 140
   black, spicy Jamaican *(Fantastic Foods* Cup), 2.4 oz. . 250
   curry, Bombay, w/lentils *(Fantastic Foods* Cup),
     2.4 oz. 250
   red *(Mahatma)* 190
   red, Cajun *(Fantastic Foods* Cup), 2.3 oz. 230
   pinto *(Mahatma)* 190
   pinto, Tex-Mex *(Fantastic Foods* Cup), 2.3 oz. 240
beef *(Success)* 190
beef or Cajun style *(Lipton* Rice & Sauce), 1 cup* 270
broccoli-cheese *(Mahatma)* 200
broccoli-cheese *(Success)* 210
brown *(Arrowhead Mills* Quick), 1/3 cup 150
brown and wild *(Arrowhead Mills* Quick), 1/4 pkg. 140
brown and wild *(Success)* 190
Cajun style, w/beans *(Lipton* Rice & Sauce), 1 cup* 310
cheddar broccoli *(Lipton* Rice & Sauce), 1 cup* 280
chicken/chicken flavor:
   (Lipton Rice & Sauce), 1 cup* 280
   (Mahatma) 190
   (Savory Classics), 1 cup* 300
   (Success Classic) 150

creamy *(Lipton* Rice & Sauce), 1 cup* 290
pilaf *(Lundberg* Quick Country) 220
chicken, roasted *(Lipton* Rice & Sauce), 1 cup* 260
chicken, southwestern *(Lipton* Rice & Sauce), 1 cup* . . . 260
chicken and broccoli *(Lipton* Rice & Sauce), 1 cup* 280
chicken and wild rice, almond *(Savory Classics),* 1 cup* . 310
curry, basmati w/lentils *(Fantastic Foods Healthy*
    Complements), ¼ cup 140
gumbo *(Mahatma)* 160
herb and butter *(Lipton* Rice & Sauce), 1 cup* 280
jambalaya *(Mahatma)* 190
long grain and wild *(Lipton* Rice & Sauce Original), 1
    cup* 280
long grain and wild *(Mahatma)* 190
long grain and wild *(Minute),* ⅓ box 230
long grain and wild *(Success)* 190
medley *(Lipton* Rice & Sauce), 1 cup* 270
Mexican *(Savory Classics* Fiesta), 1 cup* 310
Mexican, cheesy *(Old El Paso),* 2.5 oz. 250
mushroom *(Lipton* Rice & Sauce), 1 cup* 270
mushroom and herb *(Lipton* Rice & Sauce), 1 cup* 290
Oriental, stir-fry *(Lipton* Rice & Sauce), 1 cup* 270
pilaf *(Lipton* Rice & Sauce), 1 cup* 260
pilaf *(Mahatma)* 190
pilaf *(Success)* 200
pilaf, garden *(Savory Classics),* 1 cup* 240
risotto:
    (Fantastic Foods Healthy Complements Classico),
        ¼ cup 140
    chicken and Parmesan *(Lipton* Rice & Sauce),
        1 cup* 270
    Milanese *(Contadina),* ⅓ pkg. 220
    mushroom, porcini *(Contadina),* ⅓ pkg. 220
    Parmesan, creamy *(Lundberg),* ¼ cup 140
    rosemary-potato or vegetable *(Contadina),* ⅓ pkg. . . 190
    tomato-wild mushroom *(Good Harvest),* ⅓ cup 160
salsa style *(Lipton* Rice & Sauce), 1 cup* 220
scampi style *(Lipton* Rice & Sauce), 1 cup* 270
Spanish *(Fantastic Foods Healthy Complements),* ⅜ cup . 160
Spanish *(Lipton* Rice & Sauce), 1 cup* 270

Rice dishes, mix *(cont.)*
Spanish *(Mahatma)* 180
Spanish *(Old El Paso)*, 2.5 oz. 250
Spanish *(Success)* 190
teriyaki *(Lipton* Rice & Sauce), 1 cup* 270
wild rice and bean *(Good Harvest)*, ⅓ cup 160
yellow *(Mahatma)* 190
Rice pudding *(Kozy Shack)*, ½ cup 130
Rice pudding mix *(Jell-O Americana)*, ½ cup* 160
Rigatoni entree, frozen, jumbo, w/meatballs *(Lean
    Cuisine Hearty Portions)*, 15⅜ oz. 440
Risotto, see "Rice dishes, mix"
Rock candy syrup *(Trader Vic's)*, 1 fl. oz. 90
Rockfish, meat only:
raw, 4 oz. 107
baked, broiled, or microwaved, 4 oz. 137
Roe (see also "Caviar"):
raw, 1 oz. 40
raw, 1 tbsp. 22
baked, broiled, or microwaved, 4 oz. 231
Roll (see also "Biscuit"), 1 roll, except as noted:
(Arnold Bran'nola Buns) 130
brown and serve *(Pepperidge Farm* Hearth), 3 rolls . . . 150
brown and serve, club *(Pepperidge Farm)* 120
brown and serve, French *(Pepperidge Farm* 3) 240
crescent, butter *(Pepperidge Farm* Heat & Serve) 110
croissant, see "Croissant"
dill-onion *(Awrey's* Deli Rounds) 150
dinner *(Arnold Bran'nola)* 70
dinner, all varieties *(Awrey's)*, 2 rolls, 1.6 oz. 110
dinner, finger, parker house, poppy, or sesame
    (Pepperidge Farm), 3 rolls 150
dinner, potato or sesame seed *(Arnold)*, 2 rolls 110
egg, twist *(Arnold Levy* Old Country) 170
French *(Arnold* 6″) 160
French *(Pepperidge Farm)* 100
French, sourdough *(Pepperidge Farm)* 100
garlic-dill or garlic-pepper *(Awrey's* Deli Rounds) . . . 150
golden twist *(Pepperidge Farm* Heat & Serve) 110
hamburger *(Arnold* 8 Pack) 130

hamburger *(Pepperidge Farm)* 130
hoagie *(Awrey's)* 230
hoagie *(Pepperidge Farm Deli Classic/Multigrain)* 200
hot dog *(Arnold 12 oz./12 Pack)* 110
hot dog *(Pepperidge Farm/Pepperidge Farm Dijon)* . . . 140
Italian *(Arnold Savoni 8″)* 280
kaiser *(Arnold Levy Old Country)* 170
kaiser *(Awrey's)* 190
kaiser, sesame *(Arnold Sandwich)* 140
onion *(Arnold Deli)* 170
onion *(Arnold Levy Old Country)* 160
sandwich *(Pepperidge Farm Hearty)* 230
sandwich, onion *(Pepperidge Farm)* 150
sandwich, potato *(Pepperidge Farm)* 160
sandwich, sesame, soft *(Arnold)* 140
sandwich, sourdough *(Pepperidge Farm)* 170
Roll, frozen or refrigerated:
crescent *(Pillsbury),* 1-oz. roll 110
crescent *(Pillsbury Reduced Fat),* 1-oz. roll 100
dinner, wheat or white *(Pillsbury),* 1.4-oz. roll 110
Roll, sweet, see "Bun, sweet"
Roseapple, 1 oz. 7
Rosemary, dried, 1 tsp. 4
Rotini dishes, mix, 1 cup*:
w/cheese, broccoli *(Kraft Velveeta)* 400
primavera *(Lipton Pasta & Sauce)* 320
three cheese *(Lipton Pasta & Sauce)* 320
Roughy, orange, meat only:
raw, 4 oz. 143
baked, broiled, or microwaved, 4 oz. 101
Rum runner mixer, frozen* *(Bacardi),* 8 fl. oz. 140
Rutabaga:
fresh, cubed, raw, ½ cup 25
fresh, boiled, drained, ½ cup 33
canned *(Sunshine),* ½ cup 30
Rye, whole-grain *(Arrowhead Mills),* ¼ cup 160
Rye flakes, rolled *(Arrowhead Mills),* ⅓ cup 110
Rye flour *(Arrowhead Mills),* ¼ cup 100
Rye-wheat flour *(Pillsbury's Bohemian Style),* ¼ cup . . . 100

FOOD AND MEASURE   **CALORIES**

Sablefish, meat only:

raw, 4 oz. 222

baked, broiled, or microwaved, 4 oz. 284

smoked, 4 oz. 291

Safflower meal, partially defatted, 1 oz. 97

Saffron, 1 tsp. 2

Sage, ground, 1 tsp. 2

Salad dressing, 2 tbsp.:

bacon and tomato *(Kraft)* 140

bacon and tomato *(Kraft Deliciously Right* Lowfat) 60

balsamic vinaigrette *(Wish-Bone)* 60

blue cheese *(Kraft Fat Free)* 50

blue cheese *(Kraft Roka)* 90

blue cheese chunky *(Seven Seas)* 90

blue cheese, chunky *(Wish-Bone)* 170

blue cheese, chunky *(Wish-Bone* Fat Free) 35

Caesar *(Kraft)* 130

Caesar *(Seven Seas Viva)* 120

Caesar *(Wish-Bone/Wish-Bone* Classic) 110

Caesar *(Wish-Bone* Fat Free) 25

Caesar, creamy *(Wish-Bone)* 180

Caesar, garlic, roasted *(Knott's Berry Farm)* 140

Caesar, ranch *(Kraft)* 140

carrot ginger *(Cary Randall's)* 5

chicken salad, Oriental *(Knott's Berry Farm)* 130

coleslaw *(Kraft)* 150

French *(Kraft)* 120

French *(Kraft Catalina)* 140

French *(Trader Vic's)* 130

French *(Wish-Bone* Deluxe) 120

French, honey *(Kraft Catalina)* 140

French, sweet 'n spicy *(Wish-Bone)* 130

French, sweet 'n spicy *(Wish-Bone* Fat Free) 30

fruit salad *(Knott's Berry Farm)* 70

Salad dressing *(cont.)*

fruit vinaigrette *(Knott's Berry Farm)* 45
garden, zesty *(Kraft Salsa)* 70
garlic, creamy *(Kraft)* 110
garlic, creamy *(Wish-Bone* Fat Free) 40
garlic, roasted, creamy *(Wish-Bone)* 110
green goddess *(Seven Seas)* 120
herb and spices *(Seven Seas)* 120
honey Dijon *(Kraft)* 150
honey Dijon *(Kraft* Fat Free) 50
honey Dijon *(Wish-Bone* Fat Free) 45
honey mustard *(Cary Randall's)* 35
honey mustard *(Knott's Berry Farm)* 130
Italian *(Kraft* Fat Free) 10
Italian *(Kraft* House) 120
Italian *(Kraft* Presto) 140
Italian *(Kraft* Zesty/Creamy) 110
Italian *(Seven Seas Viva/Seven Seas* Creamy) 110
Italian *(Seven Seas Viva* Reduced Cal) 45
Italian *(Trader Vic's)* 80
Italian *(Wish-Bone)* 80
Italian *(Wish-Bone* Classic House) 140
Italian *(Wish-Bone Robusto)* 90
Italian, cheese, 2 *(Seven Seas)* 70
Italian, creamy *(Wish-Bone)* 110
Italian, olive oil *(Wish-Bone* Classic) 60
Javanese *(Trader Vic's)* 150
mayonnaise type, see "Mayonnaise"
Oriental *(Wish-Bone)* 70
Parmesan and onion *(Wish-Bone)* 110
Parmesan and onion *(Wish-Bone* Fat Free) 45
pepper, roasted, vinaigrette *(Cary Randall's)* 10
peppercorn, ground *(Knott's Berry Farm)* 160
pesto, hemp, vinaigrette *(Cary Randall's)* 130
poppyseed *(Knott's Berry Farm)* 120
ranch *(Kraft)* 170
ranch *(Kraft Salsa)* 130
ranch *(Seven Seas)* 150
ranch *(Wish-Bone)* 160
ranch *(Wish-Bone* Lite) 100

ranch, buttermilk or cucumber *(Kraft)* 150
ranch, peppercorn or sour cream-onion *(Kraft)* 170
raspberry vinaigrette *(Knott's Berry Farm* Low Fat) 50
red wine vinegar *(Seven Seas* Lowfat) 60
red wine vinegar and oil *(Seven Seas)* 110
red wine vinaigrette *(Wish-Bone)* 80
red wine vinaigrette *(Wish-Bone* Fat Free) 35
Russian *(Kraft)* 130
Russian *(Seven Seas Viva)* 150
Russian *(Wish-Bone)* 110
sesame w/soy *(Trader Vic's* South Pacific) 110
Thousand Island *(Kraft)* 110
Thousand Island *(Kraft* Fat Free) 45
Thousand Island w/bacon *(Kraft)* 120
tomato, sun-dried, basil *(Cary Randall's)* 10
tomato, sun-dried, vinaigrette *(Knott's Berry Farm)* 100
white wine vinaigrette *(Wish-Bone)* 60
Salad dressing mix*, 2 tbsp.:
bacon or blue cheese *(Hidden Valley)* 120
buttermilk *(Hidden Valley* Original) 110
buttermilk, farm *(Good Seasons)* 120
Caesar, gourmet *(Good Seasons)* 150
cheese garlic or garlic and herbs *(Good Seasons)* 140
honey Dijon *(Hidden Valley)* 120
honey mustard *(Good Seasons)* 150
Italian *(Good Seasons)* 140
Italian *(Good Seasons* Free) 10
Italian *(Good Seasons* Reduced Cal) 50
Italian, mild *(Good Seasons)* 150
Mexican spice *(Good Seasons)* 140
Oriental sesame *(Good Seasons)* 150
ranch *(Good Seasons)* 120
ranch *(Good Seasons* Reduced Cal) 60
ranch *(Hidden Valley* Original Milk) 120
ranch *(Hidden Valley* Original Reduced Calorie) 70
ranch, Italian *(Hidden Valley)* 140
Salad toppers (see also "Croutons"), all varieties
    (Pepperidge Farm), 1 tbsp. 35
Salami:
beer *(Oscar Mayer)*, 2 slices, 1.6 oz. 110

Salami *(cont.)*
beef *(Boar's Head)*, 2 oz. 120
beef *(Hebrew National)*, 2 oz. 170
beef *(Oscar Mayer* Machiach), 2 slices, 1.6 oz. 120
cooked *(Boar's Head)*, 2 oz. 130
cotto *(Oscar Mayer)*, 2 slices, 1.6 oz. 110
cotto, beef *(Oscar Mayer)*, 2 slices, 1.6 oz. 90
dry or hard *(Boar's Head)*, 1 oz. 110
dry or hard *(Oscar Mayer)*, 3 slices, 1 oz. 100
Genoa *(Boar's Head)*, 2 oz. 180
Genoa *(Di Lusso)*, 1 oz. 120
Genoa *(Oscar Mayer)*, 3 slices, 1 oz. 100
Salisbury steak, see "Beef dinner" and "Beef entree"
Salmon, fresh, meat only, 4 oz.:
Atlantic, farmed, raw 207
Atlantic, farmed, baked, broiled, or microwaved 234
Atlantic, wild, raw 161
Atlantic, wild, baked, broiled, or microwaved 206
Chinook, raw 204
Chinook, baked, broiled, or microwaved 262
chum, raw 136
chum, baked, broiled, or microwaved 175
coho, farmed, raw 182
coho, farmed, baked, broiled, or microwaved 202
coho, wild, raw 165
coho, wild, baked, broiled, or microwaved 158
coho, boiled, poached, or steamed 209
pink, raw 132
pink, baked, broiled, or microwaved 169
sockeye, raw 191
sockeye, baked, broiled, or microwaved 245
smoked, see "Salmon, smoked"
Salmon, canned:
chum, drained, 4 oz. 160
Norwegian fillet *(Abelvaer)*, 3 oz. 170
pink, skinless fillet *(Bumble Bee)*, ¼ cup 70
red, blueback *(Rubinstein's)*, ¼ cup 110
red sockeye, *(S&W)*, ¼ cup 110
Salmon, smoked:
Chinook, 4 oz. 133

lox or Nova *(Vita)*, 2 oz. 50
lox or Nova *(Vita)*, 3-oz. pkg. 80
pastrami style *(Ducktrap River* Spruce Point), 2 oz. 130
Salmon, smoked, spread *(Vita)*, ¼ cup, 2 oz. 180
Salmon entree, frozen, grilled, creamy dill or honey
   mustard *(Mrs. Paul's/Van de Kamp's)*, 1 fillet . . . 90
Salsa (see also "Picante sauce"), 2 tbsp.:
(Christopher Ranch) 15
all varieties *(Heluva* Good) 10
all varieties *(Muir Glen)* 10
all varieties *(Pace* Thick & Chunky) 10
all varieties *(Valley of Mexico* Fire Roasted) 10
cheese, see "Cheese dip"
Salsify:
raw *(Frieda's)*, ¾ cup, 3 oz. 70
boiled, drained, sliced, ½ cup 46
Salt (see also specific listings), ¼ tsp.:
(Morton/Morton Lite Kosher) 0
seasoned *(Lawry's)* 0
seasoned *(Morton Nature's Seasons)* . . . . <1
Salt pork, raw, 1 oz. 212
Sandwich sauce, ¼ cup, except as noted:
(Frank's RedHot Buffalo), 1 tbsp. 5
(Kraft), 1 tbsp. 50
(Manwich Original) 30
Sloppy Joe *(Del Monte* Original/Hickory) 70
Sloppy Joe *(Green Giant)* 50
Sloppy Joe *(Green Giant* w/Meat) 200
Sandwich spread (see also "Meat spread," "Sandwich
   sauce" and specific listings):
(Hellmann's), 1 tbsp. 50
(Kraft Spread & Burger Sauce), 1 tbsp. 50
Sapodilla, 1 medium, 3" × 2½" 140
Sapote:
(Frieda's), 5 oz. 190
1 medium, 11.2 oz. 301
Sardine, fresh, see "Herring"
Sardine, canned:
Atlantic, in oil, drained, 2 oz. 118
Atlantic, in oil, drained, 2 medium, 3" long 50

Sardine, canned *(cont.)*

in mustard sauce *(Underwood)*, 3¾-oz. can 180
in soy oil *(Underwood)*, 3 oz. 220
in soy oil, drained, skinless, boneless *(King Oscar)*,
　　3 pieces 120
in tomato sauce *(Del Monte)*, 2 oz., ½ fish w/sauce 80
in tomato sauce *(Underwood)*, 3¾-oz. can 180
Sauce, see specific listings
Sauerkraut:
(Claussen), ¼ cup 5
(Del Monte), 2 tbsp. 0
(Pickle Eater's Kozmic Kraut/Reduced Sodium), 2 tbsp. . . . 0
(Seneca), 2 tbsp. 5
Bavarian style *(Del Monte)*, 2 tbsp. 15
Bavarian style *(Seneca)*, 2 tbsp. 10
Sauerkraut juice *(Stokely)*, 8 fl. oz. 20
Sausage (see also specific listings), cooked, 2 links,
　　except as noted:
Andouille *(Aidell's* Cajun Brand), 3.5-oz. link 220
beef, smoked *(Oscar Mayer* Smokies), 1 link 120
beef, smoked *(Healthy Choice)*, 2 oz. 70
brown and serve *(Little Sizzlers)*, 3 links 230
brown and serve *(Little Sizzlers)*, 2 patties 190
cheese *(Oscar Mayer* Little Smokies), 6 links 180
cheese *(Oscar Mayer* Smokies), 1 link 130
chicken and apple, fresh, raw *(Aidell's)*, 2 oz. 100
chicken and apple or lemon, smoked *(Aidell's)*, 3.5-oz.
　　link 210
chicken teriyaki, fresh, raw *(Aidell's)*, 3.5-oz. link 210
chicken and turkey (see also "turkey and chicken,"
　　below):
　　curry, smoked *(Aidell's* Burmese), 3.5-oz. link 220
　　smoked *(Aidell's* New Mexico Brand), 3.5-oz. link . . . 210
　　Thai, fresh, raw *(Aidell's)*, 3.5-oz. link 200
　　Thai, smoked *(Aidell's)*, 3.5-oz. link 220
chorizo, beef, raw *(Aidell's)*, 3.5-oz. link 400
chorizo, pork, spicy *(Battistoni)*, 1 oz. 80
duck and turkey, smoked *(Aidell's)*, 3.5-oz. link 220
Italian, pork, raw *(Aidell's)*, 3.5-oz. link 230
Italian, turkey, raw *(Aidell's)*, 3.5-oz. link 190

lamb and beef, w/rosemary, fresh, raw *(Aidell's)*, 3.5-oz.
   link 220
pickled, smoked or hot *(Hormel)*, 6 links 140
pork:
   fresh, .5 oz. (1 oz. raw link) 48
   (Jones Dairy Farm All Natural Light) 130
   (Jones Dairy Farm All Natural Little Links), 3 links . . . 190
   (Little Sizzlers), 3 links 180
   (Oscar Mayer) 180
   (Tobin's First Prize Little Links) 190
   hot and spicy *(Little Sizzlers)*, 3 links 180
   light *(Jones Dairy Farm* Golden Brown) 110
   maple *(Jones Dairy Farm* Golden Brown) 190
   mild or milk *(Jones Dairy Farm* Golden Brown) 190
   spicy *(Jones Dairy Farm* Golden Brown) 190
pork, patty *(Jones Dairy Farm* All Natural), 1 patty 130
pork, patty *(Little Sizzlers)*, 2 patties 210
pork, smoked *(Ball Park)*, 4-oz. link 240
pork, smoked *(Boar's Head)*, 4.5 oz. 400
pork, smoked *(Oscar Mayer* Little Smokies), 6 links 170
pork, hot or regular *(Hillshire Farm)*, 1 link 250
pork, whiskey fennel *(Aidell's)*, 3.5-oz. link 200
pork and turkey, breakfast *(Healthy Choice)*, 2 links/
   patties 50
pork and veal, smoked, bier or hunter *(Aidell's)*, 3.5-oz.
   link 240
smoked *(Healthy Choice)*, 2 oz. 70
tomato-basil *(Healthy Choice)*, 2 oz. 70
turkey, cranberry, smoked *(Aidell's)*, 3.5-oz. link 210
turkey, scallion-herbs, fresh, raw *(Aidell's)*, 3.5-oz. link . . 200
turkey and chicken, artichoke, smoked *(Aidell's)*, 3.5-oz.
   link 180
turkey and chicken, pesto, smoked *(Aidell's)*, 3.5-oz.
   link 220
turkey and chicken w/sun-dried tomatoes and basil
   (Aidell's), 3.5-oz. link 200
"Sausage," vegetarian:
canned *(Loma Linda* Linketts), 2 links 70
canned *(Worthington Saucettes)*, 1 link 90
frozen *(Green Giant* Breakfast), 3 links 110

"Sausage," vegetarian *(cont.)*
frozen *(Green Giant* Breakfast), 2 patties 100
frozen *(Morningstar Farms* Breakfast), 2 links 60
frozen *(Morningstar Farms* Breakfast), 1 patty 70
refrigerated *(Morningstar Farms* Breakfast), 2 patties . . . 120
Sausage stick:
(Slim Jim Big Slim), 1 piece 70
beef *(Rustlers Roundup* Jerky), .22 oz. 30
beef *(Slim Jim Big Jerk)*, 1 piece 25
beef *(Slim Jim Super Jerk)*, 1 piece 35
hot *(Rustlers Roundup* Flamin' Hot), .3 oz. 40
hot red pepper *(Pemmican Tender Jerky)*, 1-oz. bag 80
mild or spicy *(Slim Jim* Cannister), 3 pieces 150
mild or spicy *(Slim Jim* Handipak), 1 box, 5 pieces 210
smoked *(Rustlers Roundup* Steak Strip), .8 oz. 60
smoked, mild or spicy *(Slim Jim)*, 1.4-oz. box 210
spicy *(Rustlers Roundup)*, .5 oz. 70
spicy *(Slim Jim* Caddy), 1 piece 50
spicy *(Slim Jim* Giant), 1 oz. 150
spicy *(Slim Jim* Super Slim), 1 piece 100
turkey, peppered *(Pemmican* Snacks), 1 oz. 60
Savory, ground, 1 tsp. 4
Scallion, see "Onion, green"
Scallop, meat only:
raw, 4 oz. 100
raw, 2 large or 5 small, 1.1 oz. 26
"Scallop," imitation, frozen, bay style *(Louis Kemp
    Scallop Delights)*, ½ cup 80
Scallop, fried, frozen *(Mrs. Paul's)*, 5.5-oz. pkg. 330
"Scallop," vegetarian, canned:
(Loma Linda Tender Bits), 6 pieces 110
(Worthington Vegetable Skallops), ½ cup 90
Scallop squash, ½ cup:
boiled, drained, sliced 14
boiled, drained, mashed 19
Scone, all fruit varieties *(Health Valley)*, 1 piece 180
Scorpion drink mixer *(Trader Vic's)*, 4 oz. 80
Scrapple *(Jones Dairy Farm)*, 2 oz. 120
Scrod, fresh, see "Cod, Atlantic"

Scup, meat only:
raw, 4 oz. 119
baked, broiled, or microwaved, 4 oz. 153
Sea bass, meat only:
raw, 4 oz. 110
baked, broiled, or microwaved, 4 oz. 141
Sea trout, meat only:
raw, 4 oz. 118
baked, broiled, or microwaved, 4 oz. 151
Seafood, see specific listings
Seafood dip (see also "Clam dip") *(Heluva* Good), 2
    tbsp. 60
Seafood sauce (see also specific listings), cocktail, ¼
    cup:
(Crosse & Blackwell) 100
(Del Monte) 100
(Sauceworks) 60
Seasoning (see also specific listings), ¼ tsp.:
(Ac'cent), ⅛ tsp. 0
(Maggi), 1 tsp. 0
Seasoning and coating mix (see also specific listings),
    ⅛ pkt.:
country *(Shake'n Bake)* 35
glaze, tangy honey or honey mustard *(Shake'n Bake)* 45
Italian herb *(Shake'n Bake)* 40
Seaweed:
agar, flakes or bar *(Eden),* 1 tbsp. 10
arame or hiziki *(Eden),* ½ cup 30
kombu *(Eden),* ½ of 7″ piece 10
nori *(Eden),* 1 sheet 10
Semolina, whole grain, ¼ cup 150
Semolina flour, mix *(Arrowhead Mills),* ½ cup 240
Sesame butter *(Roaster Fresh),* 1 oz. 168
Sesame meal, partially defatted, 1 oz. 161
Sesame paste (see also "Tahini"), from whole seeds,
    1 tbsp. 95
Sesame seasoning *(Eden),* ½ tsp. 10
Sesame seeds:
whole, brown *(Arrowhead Mills),* ¼ cup 200
whole, roasted, toasted, 1 oz. 161

kernels, decorticated *(Arrowhead Mills)*, ¼ cup 210
Shad, meat only:
raw, 4 oz. 223
baked, broiled, or microwaved, 4 oz. 286
Shallot:
fresh or stored *(Frieda's)*, 1 tbsp., 1 oz. 20
fresh or stored, chopped, 1 tbsp. 7
freeze-dried, 1 tbsp. 3
Shark, meat only, raw, 4 oz. 148
Sheepshead, meat only:
raw, 4 oz. 123
baked, broiled, or microwaved, 4 oz. 143
Shellie beans, canned, w/liquid, ½ cup 37
Shells, pasta, mix:
Alfredo, garlic *(Fantastic Foods Healthy Complements)*,
⅔ cup 210
w/cheese or cheese and bacon *(Kraft Velveeta)*, 1 cup* . . 360
w/cheese and salsa *(Kraft Velveeta)*, 1 cup* 380
white cheddar sauce *(DeBoles)*, 2.7 oz. 260
Shells, pasta, entree, frozen, 1 pkg.:
and American cheese *(Stouffer's)*, ½ of 12-oz. pkg. 260
marinara *(Healthy Choice)*, 12 oz. 390
Sherbet (see also "Sorbet"), ½ cup, except as noted:
berry rainbow *(Edy's/Dreyer's)* 130
orange, rainbow, raspberry, or tropical *(Breyers)* 120
orange, rainbow, or tropical *(Breyers)* Fat Free 110
orange, Swiss *(Edy's/Dreyer's)* 160
orange vanilla swirl or strawberry kiwi *(Edy's/Dreyer's)* . . 120
Shortening, 1 tbsp.:
(Jewel/Swiftning) 110
lard or vegetable oil 115
vegetable *(Snowdrift)* 110
vegetable, regular/butter flavor *(Crisco)* 110
Shrimp, meat only:
raw, 4 large, 1 oz. 30
boiled or steamed, 4 oz. 112
boiled or steamed, 4 large 22
Shrimp, canned, drained, 1 cup 154
"Shrimp," imitation, frozen *(Captain Jac)*, 3 jumbo,
3 oz. 90

Shrimp sauce *(Crosse & Blackwell)*, ¼ cup 110
Shrimp entree, frozen:
and angel hair pasta *(Lean Cuisine Cafe Classics)*, 10-
    oz. pkg. 290
breaded, butterfly *(Van de Kamp's)*, 7 pieces 300
breaded, popcorn *(Van de Kamp's)*, 20 pieces 270
breaded, whole *(Van de Kamp's)*, 7 pieces 240
marinara *(Healthy Choice)*, 10.5 oz. 250
and vegetables *(Healthy Choice Maria)*, 12.5 oz. 290
Shrimp sauce *(Crosse & Blackwell)*, ¼ cup 110
Sloppy Joe sauce, see "Sandwich sauce"
Smelt, rainbow, meat only:
raw, 4 oz. 110
baked, broiled, or microwaved, 4 oz. 141
Snack bar (see also "Granola and Cereal bar"), 1 bar:
all varieties *(Sweet Rewards Fat Free)* 120
brownie *(Sweet Rewards Low Fat)* 120
chocolate chip *(Sweet Rewards Low Fat)* 110
fudge, double *(Sweet Rewards Fat Free Supreme)* 100
marshmallow *(Golden Grahams Treats)* 90
Snack mix:
(Blue Diamond Beach House), 1 oz. 110
(Blue Diamond Hot House), 1 oz. 150
(Blue Diamond Smoke House), 1 oz. 140
(Cheez-It), ½ cup 140
(Chex Mix), ⅔ cup 130
(Chex Mix Bold n' Zesty), ½ cup 150
Snail, sea, see "Whelk"
Snapper, meat only:
raw, 4 oz. 113
baked, broiled, or microwaved, 4 oz. 145
Snow peas, see "Peas, edible-podded"
Soft drinks, carbonated, 8 fl. oz., except as noted:
birch beer, brown *(Canada Dry)* 110
birch beer, clear *(Canada Dry)* 100
blueberry *(Minute Maid)* 110
cactus cooler *(Canada Dry)* 100
cherry *(Crush)* 120
cherry *(Sunkist)* 130
cherry, black *(Canada Dry)* 120

Soft drinks *(cont.)*
cherry, wild *(Canada Dry)*. 100
cherry-lime *(Slice)*, 12 fl. oz. 160
cherry-spice *(Slice)*, 12 fl. oz. 150
club soda *(Canada Dry/Schweppes)* 0
cola *(Coca-Cola* Classic/Caffeine Free) 97
cola *(Pepsi/Pepsi* Caffeine Free), 12 fl. oz. 150
cola *(RC/RC* Caffeine Free) 110
cola, cherry *(Coca-Cola)* 104
cola, cherry *(RC)*. 110
cola, cherry, wild *(Pepsi)*, 12 fl. oz. 160
cola, draft *(RC)*. 120
cream *(Barq's* Red) 115
cream *(Hires)*. 120
cream *(Mug)*, 12 fl. oz. 170
cream, vanilla *(Canada Dry)* 110
(Dr Pepper/Dr Pepper Sodium Free) 100
(Dr. Slice), 12 fl. oz. 140
fruit blend/punch *(Crush* Fruity Red/Tropical Punch) 120
fruit blend/punch *(Minute Maid)* 113
fruit blend/punch *(Welch's* Tropical Punch) 130
ginger ale *(Canada Dry/Schweppes)* 80
ginger ale *(Canada Dry* Golden) 90
ginger ale, cherry *(Canada Dry)* 100
ginger ale, grape or raspberry *(Schweppes)* 90
ginger beer *(Schweppes)* 90
grape *(Crush)* 130
grape *(Fanta)* 117
grape *(Schweppes)* 120
grape, Concord *(Canada Dry)* 110
grapefruit *(Schweppes)* 100
grapefruit *(Squirt)* 100
grapefruit, lemon *(Canada Dry* Half & Half) 100
grapefruit, ruby red *(Squirt)* 120
lemon, bitter *(Canada Dry)* 100
lemon, bitter *(Schweppes)* 110
lemon, sour *(Canada Dry)* 90
lemon, sour *(Schweppes)*. 100
lemonade, see "Lemonade"
lemon-lime *(Schweppes)* 90

lemon-lime *(Slice)*, 12 fl. oz. 150
lime *(Canada Dry* Island) 120
(Mello Yello) 118
(Mountain Dew Regular/Caffeine Free), 12 fl. oz. 170
orange *(Canada Dry* Sunripe) 110
orange *(Minute Maid)* 118
orange *(Sunkist)* 130
orange *(Welch's)* 120
orange, peach, or pineapple *(Crush)* 120
peach *(Canada Dry)* 110
peach *(Sunkist)* 110
peach *(Welch's)* 130
piña colada *(Nehi)* 110
pineapple *(Canada Dry)* 100
pineapple *(Minute Maid)* 109
pineapple *(Sunkist)* 120
(RC Dr. Nehi/RC Kick) 120
(RC Upper 10) 110
root beer *(Barrelhead)* 100
root beer *(Hires)* 120
root beer *(Mug)*, 12 fl. oz. 160
seltzer, plain or flavored *(Canada Dry/Schweppes)* 0
(7Up) 100
(Slice Red), 12 fl. oz. 190
sour mixer *(Canada Dry)* 80
(Sprite) 96
strawberry *(Crush)* 110
strawberry *(Minute Maid)* 113
strawberry *(Sunkist)* 120
strawberry *(Welch's)* 120
strawberry, California *(Canada Dry)* 100
(Sundrop) 120
(Surge) 116
tonic water, plain or cranberry *(Schweppes)* 80
tonic water, plain or lime *(Canada Dry)* 90
(Wink II) 110
Sole:
fresh, see "Flatfish"
frozen *(Van de Kamp's)*, 4-oz. fillet 110

Sole entree, frozen:

au gratin *(Oven Poppers)*, 5-oz. piece 220

breaded, fillet *(Mrs. Paul's)*, 1 piece 160

stuffed, 5-oz. piece, except as noted:

    w/broccoli, cheese *(Oven Poppers)* 150

    w/crab *(Oven Poppers)* 250

    w/crab, miniatures *(Oven Poppers)*, 2-oz. piece . . 120

    w/garlic, shrimp, almonds *(Oven Poppers)* 250

    w/shrimp and lobster *(Oven Poppers)* 150

    w/spinach and cheese *(Oven Poppers)* 210

Sopressata *(Boar's Head Cinghiale Mini)*, 1 oz. 100

Sorbet (see also "Sherbet"), ½ cup, except as noted:

banana strawberry *(Häagen-Dazs)* 140

cherry cordial *(Edy's/Dreyer's)* 160

chocolate *(Columbo* Cha Cha) 100

chocolate *(Häagen-Dazs)* 120

chocolate, devil's food *(Ben & Jerry's)* 170

and ice cream, orange or raspberry *(Häagen-Dazs)* 190

lemon *(Columbo* Twist) 100

lemon *(Edy's/Dreyer's)* 140

lemon *(Häagen-Dazs* Zesty) 120

lemon swirl *(Ben & Jerry's)* 120

mango *(Häagen-Dazs)* 120

mango lime *(Ben & Jerry's)* 130

mango orange or peach *(Edy's/Dreyer's)* 120

Margarita *(Häagen-Dazs)* 130

peach *(Columbo* Retreat) 100

peach *(Häagen-Dazs* Orchard) 140

passion fruit *(Ben & Jerry's Purple Passion Fruit)* 140

raspberry *(Columbo* Jazz) 100

raspberry or raspberry lemonade *(Häagen-Dazs)* 120

raspberry kiwi *(Edy's/Dreyer's)* 130

strawberry *(Columbo* Swing) 100

strawberry *(Edy's/Dreyer's)* 120

strawberry *(Häagen-Dazs)* 130

strawberry kiwi *(Ben & Jerry's)* 140

Sorbet bar, 1 bar:

berry, wild *(Häagen-Dazs)* 90

chocolate *(Häagen-Dazs)* 80

Sorghum, whole grain, 1 cup 650

Sorghum syrup *(Arrowhead Mills)*, 1 tbsp. 60
Sorrel, see "Dock"
Soup, canned, ready-to-serve, 1 cup:
bean, 4 *(Arrowhead Mills)* 130
bean, black *(Health Valley)* 110
bean, black *(Progresso* Hearty) 170
bean, smoky *(Arrowhead Mills)* 140
bean and ham *(Campbell's Chunky)* 190
bean and ham *(Campbell's Home Cookin')* 180
bean and ham *(Progresso)* 160
bean and vegetable *(Health Valley)* 140
bean and vegetable, black bean *(Health Valley)* 110
beef barley *(Progresso)* 130
beef broth *(Swanson* Clear). 20
beef noodle *(Progresso)* 140
beef pasta *(Campbell's Chunky)* 140
beef vegetable *(Progresso* 99% Fat Free) 160
beef vegetable, country *(Campbell's Chunky)* 150
beef vegetable and rotini *(Progresso)* 130
borscht *(Manischewitz)* 80
borscht *(Manischewitz* Low Calorie) 25
borscht, w/shredded beets *(Manischewitz)* 90
chicken *(Progresso* Chickarina) 130
chicken, rotisserie seasoned *(Progresso)* 100
chicken barley *(Progresso)* 110
chicken broccoli, cheese, potato *(Campbell's Chunky)* . . . 200
chicken broth *(Arrowhead Mills)* 60
chicken broth *(Campbell's Healthy Request)* 20
chicken broth *(College Inn)* 25
chicken broth *(Health Valley)* 45
chicken broth *(Progresso)* 20
chicken broth *(Swanson)* 20
chicken broth *(Swanson Fat Free Natural Goodness)* 15
chicken broth, w/onion *(Swanson)* 25
chicken corn chowder *(Campbell's Chunky)* 250
chicken corn chowder *(Campbell's Healthy Request
  Hearty)* 150
chicken and mushroom chowder *(Campbell's Chunky)*. . . 210
chicken noodle *(Campbell's Chunky* Classic) 130
chicken noodle *(Campbell's Healthy Request)* 100

Soup, canned, ready-to-serve *(cont.)*

chicken noodle *(Campbell's Simply Home)* 80
chicken noodle *(Progresso)* 90
chicken noodle egg *(Campbell's Home Cookin')* 90
chicken pasta *(Campbell's Simply Home)* 90
chicken pasta *(Healthy Choice)* 120
chicken pasta, and mushroom *(Campbell's Chunky)* 120
chicken pasta, w/roasted garlic *(Campbell's Home
   Cookin')* 120
chicken and penne, spicy *(Progresso)* 110
chicken rice *(Campbell's Healthy Request Hearty)* 110
chicken rice *(Campbell's Home Cookin')* 100
chicken rice, w/vegetables *(Progresso)* 90
chicken rice, white/wild *(Progresso)* 100
chicken rice, white/wild *(Campbell's Simply Home)* 100
chicken rice, white/wild, savory *(Campbell's Chunky)* . . . 140
chicken and rotini *(Progresso Hearty)* 90
chicken vegetable *(Campbell's Chunky Hearty)* 90
chicken vegetable *(Campbell's Healthy Request)* 110
chicken vegetable *(Campbell's Home Cookin')* 120
chicken vegetable *(Progresso)* 90
chicken vegetable, Italian *(Campbell's Home Cookin')* . . . 130
chicken vegetable, spicy *(Campbell's Chunky)* 90
clam chowder:
   Manhattan *(Campbell's Chunky)* 130
   Manhattan *(Progresso)* 110
   New England *(Campbell's Chunky)* 240
   New England *(Campbell's Healthy Request)* 120
   New England *(Campbell's Home Cookin')* 190
   New England *(Progresso)* 190
   New England *(Progresso 99% Fat Free)* 130
clam and rotini chowder *(Progresso)* 190
corn, country, and vegetable *(Health Valley)* 70
crab, red, vegetable *(Chincoteague)* 90
egg flower *(Rice Road)* 90
escarole, in chicken broth *(Progresso)* 25
hot and sour *(Rice Road)* 90
Italian, carotene *(Health Valley)* 80
lentil *(Health Valley)* 90
lentil *(Progresso)* 140

lentil *(Progresso* 99% Fat Free) 130
lentil, red *(Arrowhead Mills)* 100
lentil, savory *(Campbell's Home Cookin')* 130
macaroni and bean *(Progresso)* 160
meatballs and pasta pearls *(Progresso)* 140
minestrone *(Arrowhead Mills)* 110
minestrone *(Campbell's Home Cookin'* Old World) 120
minestrone *(Campbell's Simply Home)* 110
minestrone *(Progresso)* 120
minestrone, beef *(Progresso)* 140
minestrone, chicken *(Progresso)* 110
minestrone, Parmesan *(Progresso)* 100
minestrone, Tuscany *(Campbell's Home Cookin')* 190
mushroom, cream of *(Campbell's Home Cookin')* 80
mushroom broth *(Arrowhead Mills)* 10
mushroom barley *(Arrowhead Mills)* 70
mushroom barley *(Health Valley)* 60
mushroom chicken, creamy *(Progresso* 99% Fat Free) . . . 90
mushroom rice, country *(Campbell's Home Cookin')* 90
noodles, Oriental, vegetable *(Campbell's Home Cookin')* . 100
onion, creamy *(Arrowhead Mills)* 100
Oriental broth *(Swanson)* 15
pasta, Bolognese, cacciatore, or Romano *(Health Valley)* . 100
pasta, Chinese *(Rice Road)* 70
pasta, fagioli *(Health Valley)* 120
pasta, primavera *(Health Valley)* 110
pasta, roasted garlic, lentil *(Progresso)* 120
pea, split *(Health Valley)* 110
pea, split *(Progresso* 99% Fat Free) 170
pea, split, w/bacon *(Grandma Brown's)* 210
pea, split, green *(Progresso)* 170
pea, split, w/ham *(Campbell's Chunky)* 190
pea, split, w/ham *(Campbell's Healthy Request)* 170
pea, split, w/ham *(Campbell's Home Cookin')* 170
pea, split, w/ham *(Progresso)* 150
penne, in chicken broth *(Progresso* Hearty) 80
penne, oregano, Italian style vegetable *(Progresso)* 90
penne, peppercorn vegetable *(Progresso)* 100
pepper steak *(Campbell's Chunky)* 130

Soup, canned, ready-to-serve *(cont.)*
potato, baked:
   w/bacon bits, chives *(Campbell's Chunky)* 170
   w/cheddar, bacon bits *(Campbell's Chunky)* 180
   w/steak, cheese *(Campbell's Chunky)* 200
potato, broccoli and cheese *(Progresso)* 160
potato, creamy, w/roasted garlic *(Campbell's Healthy*
   Request) 110
potato, w/roasted garlic *(Campbell's Home Cookin')* 180
potato, ham and cheese *(Progresso)* 170
potato, white cheddar *(Progresso 99% Fat Free)* 140
potato ham chowder *(Campbell's Chunky Old*
   Fashioned) 220
potato leek *(Health Valley)* 70
rotini, herb, vegetable *(Progresso)* 120
rotini, tomato, basil *(Progresso)* 120
rotini and vegetable *(Health Valley Pasta Soup)* 100
sirloin burger w/vegetable *(Campbell's Chunky)* 210
steak and potato *(Campbell's Chunky)* 150
tomato *(Campbell's)* 100
tomato *(Health Valley)* 90
tomato *(Muir Glen)* 60
tomato *(Progresso/Progresso Hearty/Basil)* 100
tomato, creamy *(Campbell's)* 130
tomato, black bean *(Muir Glen)* 100
tomato, garden *(Campbell's Home Cookin')* 100
tomato, minestrone or rice *(Muir Glen)* 80
tomato vegetable *(Arrowhead Mills)* 90
tomato vegetable *(Progresso)* 90
tomato vegetable, garden *(Progresso 99% Fat Free)* 100
tomato vegetable, ravioli *(Campbell's Chunky)* 150
tortellini, cheese, w/chicken, vegetables *(Campbell's*
   Chunky) 110
tortellini, cheese and herb, tomato *(Progresso Pasta*
   Soups) 140
tortellini in chicken broth *(Progresso)* 70
turkey noodle *(Progresso)* 90
turkey rice, w/vegetables *(Progresso)* 110
vegetable *(Campbell's Chunky)* 130
vegetable *(Campbell's Healthy Request Hearty)* 100

vegetable *(Campbell's Home Cookin'* Fiesta) 140
vegetable *(Health Valley)* 80
vegetable *(Progresso)* 90
vegetable *(Progresso* 99% Fat Free) 70
vegetable, country *(Campbell's Home Cookin')* 110
vegetable, garden *(Campbell's Simply Home)* 110
vegetable, w/pasta *(Campbell's Chunky* Hearty) 140
vegetable, Southwestern *(Campbell's Healthy Request)* . . 140
vegetable barley *(Health Valley)* 90
vegetable beef *(Campbell's Chunky* Old Fashioned) 150
vegetable beef *(Campbell's Healthy Request* Hearty) . . . 140
vegetable beef *(Campbell's Home Cookin')* 110
vegetable beef, w/pasta *(Campbell's Simply Home)* 120
vegetable broth *(Arrowhead Mills)* 15
vegetable broth *(Swanson* Clear) 20
Soup, canned, condensed, undiluted, ½ cup:
asparagus, cream of *(Campbell's)* 90
barley and mushroom *(Manischewitz)* 100
bean, black *(Campbell's)* 110
bean w/bacon *(Campbell's)* 180
bean and ham, w/bacon *(Campbell's Healthy Request)* . . . 150
beef broth, double rich *(Campbell's)* 15
beef consomme *(Campbell's)* 25
beef noodle *(Campbell's)* 70
beef w/vegetables and barley *(Campbell's)* 80
broccoli, cream of *(Campbell's)* 100
broccoli, cream of *(Campbell's* 98% Fat Free) 80
broccoli, *(Campbell's Healthy Request)* 70
broccoli cheese *(Campbell's)* 110
broccoli cheese, cream of *(Campbell's* 98% Fat Free) . . . 80
celery, cream of *(Campbell's)* 110
celery, cream of *(Campbell's* 98% Fat Free) 80
celery, cream of *(Campbell's Healthy Request)* 70
cheese, cheddar *(Campbell's)* 90
cheese, nacho *(Campbell's* Fiesta) 140
chicken:
    alphabet, w/vegetables *(Campbell's)* 80
    broth *(Campbell's)* 30
    broth *(Manischewitz)* 15
    cream of *(Campbell's)* 130

Soup, canned, condensed, chicken *(cont.)*
　cream of *(Campbell's 98% Fat Free)* 80
　cream of *(Campbell's Healthy Request)* 70
　cream of, and broccoli *(Campbell's)* 120
　cream of, w/herbs *(Campbell's)* 80
　dumplings *(Campbell's)* 80
　gumbo *(Campbell's)* 60
　w/kreplach *(Manischewitz)* 35
　w/matzo balls *(Manischewitz)* 80
　noodle *(Campbell's)* 70
　noodle *(Campbell's* Homestyle) 70
　noodle *(Campbell's Healthy Request)* 70
　noodle *(Campbell's Noodle O's)* 80
　noodle *(Manischewitz)* 35
　noodle, creamy *(Campbell's)* 130
　noodle, curly *(Campbell's)* 80
　mushroom, cream of *(Campbell's)* 130
　rice *(Campbell's)* 70
　w/rice *(Campbell's Healthy Request)* 60
　and stars *(Campbell's)* 70
　vegetable *(Campbell's)* 80
　vegetable *(Campbell's Healthy Request)* 80
　vegetable, Southwestern *(Campbell's)* 110
　w/white and wild rice *(Campbell's)* 70
chili beef w/beans *(Campbell's* Fiesta) 170
clam chowder:
　Manhattan *(Campbell's)* 60
　Manhattan *(Chincoteague)* 100
　New England *(Campbell's)* 90
　New England *(Campbell's 98% Fat Free)* 90
　New England *(Cape Cod* Premium 99% Fat Free) 60
　New England *(Chincoteague)* 80
corn chowder *(Chincoteague)* 100
crab, cream of *(Chincoteague)* 200
lentil *(Manischewitz)* 140
lobster bisque *(Chincoteague)* 90
minestrone *(Campbell's)* 90
mushroom:
　beefy *(Campbell's)* 70
　cream of *(Campbell's)* 110

cream of *(Campbell's/Campbell's Healthy Request)*. . . . 70
cream of, w/roasted garlic *(Campbell's)* 70
golden *(Campbell's)* 80
noodle, double, in chicken broth *(Campbell's)* 100
noodle and ground beef *(Campbell's)* 100
noodle stars, super *(Campbell's)* 50
onion, cream of *(Campbell's)* 110
onion, French *(Campbell's)* 70
oyster stew *(Campbell's)* 90
pea, green or split w/ham *(Campbell's)* 180
pepperpot *(Campbell's)* 100
potato, cream of *(Campbell's)* 90
Scotch broth *(Campbell's)* 80
shrimp, cream of *(Campbell's)* 100
tomato *(Campbell's)* 80
tomato *(Campbell's Healthy Request)* 90
tomato, Italian, w/basil, oregano *(Campbell's)* 100
tomato bisque *(Campbell's)* 130
tomato rice *(Campbell's Old Fashioned)* 120
turkey noodle *(Campbell's)* 80
turkey vegetable *(Campbell's)* 80
vegetable *(Campbell's)* 80
vegetable *(Campbell's Old Fashioned)* 70
vegetable *(Campbell's Healthy Request)* 90
vegetable, California style *(Campbell's)* 60
vegetable, hearty, w/pasta *(Campbell's)* 90
vegetable, vegetarian *(Campbell's)* 90
wonton *(Campbell's)* 45
Soup, frozen:
clam chowder *(Marie Callender's)*, 13.5 oz. 590
corn chowder *(Cascadian Farm Veggie Bowl)*, 9 oz. 170
Soup mix, dry, 1 pkg., except as noted:
asparagus, creamy *(Fantastic Foods Cup)* 130
asparagus, creamy *(Maggi)*, 1/4 pkg. 60
bean:
    black *(Fantastic Foods Jumpin' Hearty Cup)* 210
    black *(Manischewitz Instant)* 200
    black, spicy, w/couscous *(Health Valley)*, 1/3 cup . . . 130
    black, zesty, w/rice *(Health Valley)*, 1/3 cup 100
    five *(Fantastic Foods Hearty Cup)* 230

Soup mix, bean *(cont.)*

four *(Manischewitz)*, ⅕ pkg. 110
lima w/barley *(Manischewitz)*, ⅙ pkg. 80
bean, w/bacon and ham *(Campbell's* Microwave) 180
beef noodle *(Maggi)*, ¼ pkg. 50
broccoli cheddar *(Fantastic Foods* Cup) 160
broccoli cheese *(Cup-a-Soup)* 70
chicken:
    broth *(Cup-a-Soup)* 20
    broth w/pasta *(Cup-a-Soup)* 45
    country, w/pasta and herbs *(Lipton Soup Secrets
        Kettle Style)*, 1 cup* 100
    cream of *(Cup-a-Soup)* 70
    creamy *(Maggi)*, ¼ pkg. 60
    noodle *(Campbell's* Microwave) 90
    noodle *(Campbell's* Soup & Recipe), 3 tbsp. 90
    noodle *(Cup-a-Soup)* 50
    noodle *(Maggi)*, ¼ pkg. 50
    noodle *(Manischewitz* Instant) 140
    noodle, double *(Campbell's* Soup & Recipe) 170
    noodle, hearty *(Cup-a-Soup)* 60
    noodle, w/white chicken meat *(Lipton* Soup Mix),
        3 tbsp. 80
    and onion *(Lipton Soup Secrets Kettle Style)*, 1 cup* . 120
    w/pasta and beans *(Lipton Soup Secrets Kettle
        Style)*, 1 cup* 110
    rice *(Campbell's* Microwave) 120
    rice *(Manischewitz* Instant) 130
    seashell *(Maggi)*, ¼ pkg. 50
chili *(Fantastic Cha-Cha* Hearty Cup) 220
corn chowder and potato, creamy *(Fantastic Foods* Cup) . 170
couscous w/lentil *(Fantastic Foods* Hearty Cup) 230
garlic mushroom, creamy *(Fantastic Foods* Cup) 160
herb, fiesta, w/red pepper *(Lipton Recipe Secrets)*,
    1 cup* 30
herb, golden, w/lemon *(Lipton Recipe Secrets)*, 1 cup* . . . 35
herb, Italian, w/tomato *(Lipton Recipe Secrets)*, 1 cup* . . . 40
herb, savory, w/garlic *(Lipton Recipe Secrets)*, 1 cup* . . . 30
lentil *(Fantastic Foods* Country Hearty Cup) 230
lentil, hearty *(Manischewitz)* 140

lentil, w/bow-ties *(Lipton Soup Secrets Kettle Style),*
1 cup* 130
lentil, w/couscous *(Health Valley),* ⅓ cup 130
matzo ball *(Manischewitz* Instant) 40
minestrone *(Fantastic Foods* Hearty Cup) 150
minestrone *(Lipton Soup Secrets Kettle Style),* 1 cup* . . . 110
minestrone *(Manischewitz* Instant) 210
mushroom, beefy *(Lipton Recipe Secrets),* 1½ tbsp. 35
mushroom, creamy *(Cup-a-Soup)* 60
noodle, chicken free *(Fantastic* Ramen Cup) 140
noodle, onion and Oriental *(Sanwa* Ramen), ½ block . . 180
noodle, ring *(Cup-a-Soup)* 50
noodle, beef *(Campbell's* Baked Ramen), ½ block 140
noodle, beef *(Campbell's* Fried Ramen) 290
noodle, beef *(Campbell's* Low Fat Ramen) 210
noodle, beef *(Campbell's/Sanwa* Raman), ½ block 170
noodle, chicken *(Campbell's* Baked Ramen), ½ block . . . 140
noodle, chicken *(Campbell's* Low Fat Ramen) 210
noodle, chicken, w/broth *(Lipton* Soup Mix), 2 tbsp. 60
noodle, chicken, w/broth *(Lipton Ring-O-Noodle),*
2 tbsp. 70
noodle, chicken, w/real broth *(Campbell's* Quality),
3 tbsp. 100
noodle, chicken, spicy *(Campbell's* Baked Ramen),
½ block 140
noodle, chicken, spicy *(Campbell's/Sanwa* Ramen), ½
block 170
noodle, Oriental *(Campbell's* Low Fat Ramen) 220
noodle, Oriental *(Campbell's* Low Fat Ramen), ½ block . . 140
noodle, oriental *(Campbell's/Sanwa* Ramen), ½ block . . . 170
noodle, pork *(Campbell's* Ramen), ½ block 170
noodle, shrimp *(Campbell's* Fried Ramen), ½ block 170
noodle, vegetable curry *(Fantastic Foods* Ramen Cup) . . . 140
noodle, vegetable, miso *(Fantastic Foods* Ramen Cup) . . . 130
noodle, vegetable, tomato *(Fantastic Foods* Ramen Cup) . 150
onion *(Campbell's* Soup & Recipe), 1 tbsp. 20
onion *(Lipton Recipe Secrets),* 1 tbsp. 20
onion *(Mrs. Grass* Soup/Recipe), ¼ pkg. 35
onion, beefy *(Lipton Recipe Secrets),* 1 tbsp. 25
onion, golden *(Lipton Recipe Secrets),* 1⅔ tbsp. 50

Soup mix *(cont.)*

onion, mushroom *(Lipton Recipe Secrets)*, 1²/₃ tbsp. 30
onion, mushroom *(Mrs. Grass* Soup/Recipe), ¼ pkg. 60
pasta, spiral, w/chicken broth *(Lipton* Soup Mix),
   3 tbsp. 60
pea, green *(Cup-a-Soup)* 80
pea, snow, cream of *(Knorr* Chef's), 3 tbsp. 70
pea, split *(Fantastic* Hearty Cup) 190
pea, split, w/barley *(Manischewitz)*, ⅕ pkg. 110
pea, split, garden, w/carrots *(Health Valley)*, ½ cup 130
potato, creamy *(Maggi)*, ¼ pkg. 70
potato, w/broccoli *(Health Valley)*, ⅓ cup 70
potato leek, creamy *(Fantastic Foods* Cup) 120
rice and beans, Mexican *(Campbell's Soupsations)* 210
seafood, creamy *(Maggi)*, ¼ pkg. 80
spicy *(Maggi* Thick n Spicy), ½ pkg. 110
tomato *(Cup-a-Soup)* 100
vegetable *(Lipton Recipe Secrets)*, 1²/₃ tbsp. 30
vegetable, chicken flavor *(Cup-a-Soup)* 50
vegetable, chicken flavor, creamy *(Cup-a-Soup)* 80
vegetable, w/mushrooms *(Manischewitz)*, ⅕ pkg. 120
vegetable, spring *(Cup-a-Soup)* 45
vegetable barley *(Fantastic Foods* Hearty Cup) 150
vegetable beef *(Campbell's* Microwave) 90
Soup base, mix, ⅛ pkg., except as noted:
beef, ground, vegetable *(Wyler's Soup Starter)* 80
beef barley vegetable *(Wyler's Soup Starter)* 100
beef stew, hearty *(Wyler's Stew Starter)* 60
beef vegetable *(Wyler's Soup Starter)* 90
chicken noodle *(Wyler's Soup Starter)* 80
chicken vegetable, hearty *(Wyler's Soup Starter)*,
   ⅐ pkg. 70
chicken w/white and wild rice *(Wyler's Soup Starter)* 70
Sour cream, see "Cream, sour"
Soursop, ½ cup 75
Soy beverage, 8 fl. oz.:
(Soy Dream Original) 140
(Soy Moo Fat Free) 110
carob or chocolate *(Soy Dream)* 210
vanilla *(Soy Dream)* 170

vanilla *(Soy Dream* Enriched) 160
Soy flour *(Arrowhead Mills),* ½ cup 200
Soy milk, see "Soy beverage"
Soy sauce, 1 tbsp.:
(Kikkoman/Kikkoman Lite) 10
(La Choy) 10
(La Choy Lite) 15
Polynesian *(Trader Vic's)* 10
Soybean, ½ cup:
green, boiled, drained 127
dried, raw *(Arrowhead Mills),* ¼ cup 170
dried, boiled 149
dried, dry-roasted 387
dried, roasted 405
Soybean cake or curd, see "Tofu"
Soybean kernels, roasted, toasted, 1 oz. or 95 kernels . . 129
Spaghetti, dry, see "Pasta"
Spaghetti dishes, mix:
w/meat sauce *(Kraft* Dinner), 5.5 oz. 330
mild or tangy *(Kraft* American Dinner), 2 oz. 200
Spaghetti entree, canned, 1 cup:
w/franks *(Franco-American SpaghettiO's)* 250
w/meatballs *(Franco-American SpaghettiO's/Superiore)* . . 260
in tomato and cheese *(Franco-American SpaghettiO's)* . . . 190
Spaghetti entree, frozen:
marinara w/cheese garlic bread *(Marie Callender's),*
    1 cup and 2 oz. bread 410
w/meat sauce *(Lean Cuisine),* 11½-oz. pkg. 290
w/meat sauce *(Stouffer's),* 10-oz. pkg. 350
w/meat sauce, and garlic bread *(Marie Callender's),*
    1 cup and 2 oz. bread 360
w/meatballs *(Lean Cuisine),* 9½-oz. pkg. 280
w/meatballs *(Stouffer's),* 12⅝-oz. pkg. 440
and sauce, w/seasoned beef *(Healthy Choice),* 10-oz.
    pkg. 280
Spaghetti sauce, see "Pasta sauce"
Spaghetti squash:
raw *(Frieda's),* ¾ cup, 3 oz. 30
baked or boiled, drained, ½ cup 23
Spareribs, see "Pork"

Spelt flour *(Arrowhead Mills)*, ¼ cup 100
Spinach, fresh, ½ cup:
raw, chopped 6
boiled, drained 21
Spinach, canned, ½ cup:
(Allens Popeye) 45
(Allens Popeye Low Sodium) 35
(Del Monte) 30
chopped *(Allens Popeye/Sunshine)* 40
Spinach, frozen (see also "Spinach dishes"):
(Green Giant), ¾ cup 25
(Green Giant Harvest Fresh), ½ cup 25
leaf *(Seabrook)*, 1 cup 20
chopped *(Cascadian Farm)*, ⅓ cup 20
in butter sauce, cut *(Green Giant)*, ½ cup 40
Spinach, New Zealand, chopped:
raw, 1 oz. or ½ cup 4
boiled, drained, ½ cup 11
Spinach, water *(Frieda's* Ong Choy), 2 cups, 3 oz. 20
Spinach dishes, frozen:
creamed *(Green Giant)*, ½ cup 80
creamed *(Seabrook)*, ½ cup 120
creamed *(Stouffer's* Side Dish), ½ cup, 4.5 oz. 160
Indian *(Deep* Palak Paneer), 5 oz. 230
souffle *(Stouffer's* Side Dish), ½ cup, 4 oz. 150
Spinach entree, packaged, w/rice, 1 pkg.:
w/cheese *(Tamarind Tree)* Palak Paneer) 380
w/garbanzos *(Tamarind Tree* Saag Chole) 370
Spinach Masala sauce, cooking *(Shahi* Indian Magic),
¼ cup 40
Spinach-artichoke dip *(Classy Delights)*, 2 tbsp. 25
Spinach-feta pocket, frozen *(Amy's)*, 4.5 oz. piece 200
Spinach-feta appetizer, frozen:
(Cohen's), 5 pieces, 3 oz. 220
(The Fillo Factory), 5 pieces, 5 oz. 360
Spinach-feta snack *(Amy's)*, 6 pieces 160
Spiny lobster, meat only:
raw, 4 oz. 127
boiled or steamed, 2-lb. lobster w/shell 233
boiled or steamed, 4 oz. 138

Spirals, pasta, mix, 4 cheese *(Fantastic Foods Healthy Complements)*, ²⁄₃ cup 210
Split peas:
boiled, ½ cup 116
green, dry *(Arrowhead Mills)*, ¼ cup 170
Sports drink, 8 fl. oz., except as noted:
(Powerade Jagged Ice/Mountain Blast) 73
all flavors *(All Sport)* 70
fruit punch, lemon-lime and *Tidal Burst (Powerade)* 72
orange tangerine *(Powerade)* 71
Spot, meat only:
raw, 4 oz. 140
baked, broiled, or microwaved, 4 oz. 179
Sprouts (see also specific listings):
canned *(La Choy)*, 1 cup 10
stir-fry *(Frieda's)*, 1 cup 15
spicy *(Frieda's)*, 1 cup 10
Squab, fresh, raw:
meat w/skin, 4 oz. 333
breast meat only, 4 oz. 161
Squash (see also specific squash listings), frozen, winter *(Cascadian Farm)*, ½ cup 50
Squid, meat only, raw, 4 oz. 104
St. Honore, frozen dessert *(Manzoni)*, 3.5 oz. 290
Star fruit, see "Carambola"
Steak, see "Beef"
Steak sauce, 1 tbsp., except as noted:
(Crosse & Blackwell) 30
(Heinz 57) 15
(HP) 15
(Hunt's) 10
(Peter Luger Steak House) 30
(Texas Best) 15
(Trappey's Great American) 16
and burger *(Try Me Bullfighter)* 15
Caribbean *(Tabasco)* 15
garlic peppercorn or sweet-spicy *(Lea & Perrins)* 25
New Orleans style *(Tabasco)* 15
New Orleans style *(Trappey's Chef-Magic)* 10
peppercorn *(Lawry's Weekday Gourmet)*, 2 tbsp. 40

Stir-fry sauce (see also "Marinade," and specific listings), 1 tbsp.:
(Ka•Me) 10
(Ken's Steak House) 20
(Kikkoman) 15
(Lawry's) 25
garlic and ginger *(Rice Road)* 25
honey *(Ken's Steak House)* 20
lemon *(Rice Road)* 15
and rib, garlic *(Mi-Kee)* 30
teriyaki *(Rice Road)* 20
Stomach, pork, raw, 1 oz. 44
Strawberry:
fresh, ½ cup 23
canned in heavy syrup, ½ cup 117
frozen *(Cascadian Farm)*, 1 cup 90
Strawberry, dried *(Frieda's)*, ½ cup, 1.4 oz. 150
Strawberry drink:
(Capri Sun Cooler), 6.75 fl. oz. 100
nectar *(Kern's)*, 8 fl. oz. 150
nectar *(Libby's/Kern's)*, 11.5 fl. oz. 210
Strawberry drink blends, 8 fl. oz.:
(Fruitopia Strawberry Passion Awareness) 114
kiwi *(Tropicana Twister)* 130
kiwi *(V8 Splash)* 110
orange *(Season's Best)* 130
Strawberry syrup, 2 tbsp., except as noted:
(Hershey's) 100
(Knott's Berry Farm) 120
(Smucker's), ¼ cup 210
(Smucker's Light), ¼ cup 130
(Smucker's Sundae) 110
Strawberry topping, 2 tbsp.:
(Kraft) 110
(Smucker's) 100
Strawberry-peach-banana smoothie *(Del Monte* Blenders), 6.25 fl. oz. 180
String beans, see "Green bean"
Strudel, apple *(Entenmann's)*, ¼ strudel 320

Stroganoff mix (see also "Tofu dishes, mix"),
vegetarian *(Natural Touch)*, 4 tbsp. 90
Stuffing *(Arnold* Unspiced/Cornbread), 2 cups 250
Stuffing mix, dry:
(Kellogg's Crouettes), 1 cup 120
all varieties *(Stove Top)*, ⅙ box 110
chicken flavor *(Stove Top* Flexible Serving), ½ cup 120
chicken flavor *(Stove Top* Microwave), ⅙ box 130
corn bread *(Stove Top* Flexible Serving), ½ cup 110
corn bread, homestyle *(Stove Top* Microwave), ⅙ box . . . 120
herb *(Stove Top* Flexible Serve), 1 oz. 120
Sturgeon, meat only:
raw, 4 oz. 120
baked, broiled, or microwaved, 4 oz. 153
smoked, 4 oz. 196
Succotash, ½ cup:
canned kernel *(Seneca)* 90
canned, cream-style corn 102
frozen, boiled, drained 79
Sucker, white, meat only:
raw, 4 oz. 105
baked, broiled, or microwaved, 4 oz. 135
Sugar, beet or cane:
brown, 1 oz. 107
granulated, 1 tbsp. 46
granulated, 1 tsp. 15
powdered or confectioner's, 1 tbsp., unsifted 31
Sugar, maple, 1 oz. 99
Sugar, substitute:
(Equal), 1 pkt. 4
(NutraSweet), 1 tsp. 2
Sugar apple, 1 medium, 9.9 oz. 146
Sugar snap peas, see "Peas, edible-podded"
Summer sausage *(Oscar Mayer)*, 2 slices, 1.6 oz. 140
Sunfish, pumpkin-seed, meat only:
raw, 4 oz. 101
baked, broiled, or microwaved, 4 oz. 129
Sunflower seed:
(Frito-Lay), 1 oz. 180
dried, hulled *(Arrowhead Mills)*, ¼ cup 180

Sunflower seed *(cont.)*
dry-roasted *(River Queen)*, ¼ cup, 1.1 oz. 170
dry-roasted *(River Queen* Unsalted)*, ¼ cup, 1.2 oz. 200
Sunflower seed butter, 1 tbsp. 93
Swamp cabbage:
raw, .6-oz. shoot 2
boiled, drained, chopped, ½ cup 10
Sweet dumpling squash *(Frieda's)*, ¾ cup, 3 oz. 30
Sweet peas, see "Peas, green"
Sweet potato:
raw, 5″ × 2″ potato 136
baked in skin 5″ × 2″ potato 118
baked in skin, mashed, ½ cup 103
boiled w/out skin, mashed, ½ cup 172
Sweet potato, canned, ½ cup, except as noted:
whole *(Royal Prince/Trappey's)*, 4 pieces 200
halves *(Royal Prince)*, 5.7 oz., 3 pieces 190
cut or pieces *(Allens/Sugary Sam/Princella* Yams),
   ⅔ cup 160
mashed *(Princella/Sugary Sam)*, ⅔ cup 120
candied or orange-pineapple *(Royal Prince)* 210
Sweet potato, frozen, baked, cubed, ½ cup 88
Sweet and sour sauce, 2 tbsp., except as noted:
(Contadina) 40
(Kikkoman) 35
(Kraft) 80
(Sauceworks) 60
(World Harbors Maui Mountain) 60
chicken *(Gold's Dip'n Joy)*, 1 tbsp. 30
duck sauce *(Ka•Me)* 80
duck sauce, all varieties *(Gold's)* 60
Sweetbreads, see "Pancreas" and "Thymus"
Swiss chard, fresh:
raw *(Frieda's)*, 1 cup, 3 oz. 15
raw, chopped, ½ cup 3
boiled, drained, chopped, ½ cup 18
Swordfish, fresh, meat only:
raw, 4 oz. 137

baked, broiled, or microwaved, 4 oz. 176
Syrup, see specific listings
Szechwan sauce (see also "Stir-fry sauce"):
(Ka•Me), 1 tbsp. 25
cooking *(Kylin* Chili & Tomato), ¼ cup 50

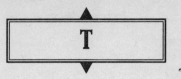

T

FOOD AND MEASURE   **CALORIES**

Tabouli *(Yorgo* Salad), 2 tbsp. 25
Taco Bell, 1 serving:
breakfast items:
    burrito, double bacon and egg 480
    burrito, country 270
    burrito, fiesta 280
    burrito, grande 420
    hash brown nuggets 280
burritos:
    bean 380
    BIG BEEF Supreme 520
    BIG CHICKEN Supreme 500
    burrito supreme 440
    chili cheese 330
    grilled chicken 400
    7-layer 530
Fajita Wrap, chicken 460
Fajita Wrap, steak 470
Fajita Wrap, veggie 420
Fajita Wrap Supreme, chicken 520
Fajita Wrap Supreme, steak 510
Fajita Wrap Supreme, veggie 510
gorditas:
    Supreme, beef or grilled chicken 300
    Supreme, steak 310
    Fiesta, beef 290
    Fiesta, grilled chicken 260
    Fiesta, steak 270
    Santa Fe, beef 380
    Santa Fe, grilled chicken or steak 370
taco, regular 180
taco, double decker 340
taco, soft 220
taco, soft, grilled chicken 200

Taco Bell (cont.)
taco, grilled steak 230
Taco Supreme, regular 220
Taco Supreme, double decker 390
Taco Supreme, soft 260
Taco Supreme, soft, grilled steak 290
specialties:
   BIG BEEF MexiMelt 290
   Mexican pizza 570
   taco salad, w/salsa 850
   taco salad, w/salsa, w/out shell 420
   tostada 300
   quesadilla, cheese 350
   quesadilla, chicken 410
nachos and sides:
   BIG BEEF nacho supreme 450
   nachos 320
   nachos *BellGrande* 770
   Pintos 'n cheese or Mexican rice 190
   twists, cinnamon 140
ice cream dessert, *Choco Taco* 310
Taco dinner mix, dry, except as noted:
(El Rio Kit), ⅕ pkg. 130
(Old El Paso Kit), 2 tacos* 330
(Ortega Kit), ⅙ pkg. 150
(Pancho Villa Kit), 2 tacos* 360
soft *(Old El Paso* Kit), 2 tacos* 400
soft *(Ortega* Kit), ⅕ pkg. 240
Taco sauce, 1 tbsp.:
all varieties *(Old El Paso/Old El Paso* Chunky) 5
green *(La Victoria)* 0
red *(La Victoria)* 5
Taco seasoning mix:
(Old El Paso), 2 tsp. 20
(Old El Paso 40% Less Sodium), 2 tsp. 15
(Pancho Villa), 2 tsp. 20
cheesy *(Old El Paso),* 1 tbsp. 15
Taco shell (see also "Tortilla"):
(Old El Paso), 3 shells 150
(Old El Paso Super), 2 shells 170

(Pancho Villa), 3 shells 160
mini *(Old El Paso)*, 7 shells 150
tostada *(Old El Paso)*, 3 shells 150
white corn *(Old El Paso)*, 3 shells 150
Tagliatelle, refrigerated, spinach *(Contadina)*, 1¼ cup . . . 270
Tahini *(Arrowhead Mills)*, 2 tbsp. 190
Tamale, canned:
(Van Camp's), 2 pieces 210
in gravy *(Old El Paso)*, 3 pieces 320
Tamale pocket, frozen *(Amy's)*, 4.5-oz. piece 250
Tamale pot pie, frozen, Mexican *(Amy's)*, 8 oz. 220
Tamarillo, 2 pieces, 4.2 oz.:
red *(Frieda's)* 40
yellow *(Frieda's)* 30
Tamarind, 1 fruit, 3″ × 1″ 5
Tandoori paste, mild *(Patak's)*, 2 tbsp. 30
Tangerine:
fresh, 1 medium, 2⅜″ 37
fresh, sections w/out membrane, ½ cup 43
canned, in light syrup *(Del Monte* Mandarin), ½ cup 80
Tangerine drink, 8 fl. oz.:
(Fruitopia Tremendously Tangerine) 109
(Mandarin Magic) 120
Tangerine juice, 8 fl. oz.:
frozen* *(Minute Maid* Beverage) 120
blend *(Dole* Mandarin) 140
blend *(Tropicana Pure Premium)* 110
Tapioca (see also "Pudding"), dry *(Minute)*, 1½ tsp. 20
Taro, cooked, sliced, ½ cup 94
Taro chips, 1 oz. 141
Taro, Tahitian, cooked, sliced, ½ cup 30
Tarragon, ground, 1 tsp. 5
Tart, snack, all varieties *(Health Valley* Healthy), 1 piece . 150
Tart shell, see "Pastry shell"
Tartar sauce, 2 tbsp.:
(Hellmann's/Best Foods) 140
(Kraft Nonfat) 25
(Sauceworks) 100
lemon herb flavor *(Sauceworks)* 150
Tartufo, frozen *(Manzoni)*, 3 oz. 200

TCBY, all flavors, ½ cup:
hand-dipped, ice cream, regular 140
hand-dipped, ice cream, lowfat, no sugar, or nonfat 100
hand-dipped, yogurt, frozen, 96% fat free 110
hand-dipped, yogurt, frozen, nonfat 100
soft serve, sorbet 100
soft-serve, yogurt, frozen, 96% fat free 140
soft-serve, yogurt, frozen, nonfat 110
soft-serve, yogurt, frozen, nonfat, no sugar 80
Tea (see also "Tea, iced"), 1 bag or 1 tsp.:
plain, regular or instant, all varieties 0
flavored, lemon, instant *(Lipton)* 0
Tea, iced, 8 fl. oz., except as noted:
(Hood) 100
(Nestea) 63
(Nestea Cool) 82
(Schweppes) 90
(Snapple) 70
all fruit flavors *(Lipton* Chilled) 80
lemon *(Nestea)* 77
lemon *(Snapple)* 100
lemon *(Tropicana)* 100
mango or passion fruit *(Snapple)* 110
mint *(Snapple)* 120
peach *(Nestea)* 78
peach or raspberry *(Tropicana),* 11.5 fl. oz. 160
peach, raspberry, or strawberry *(Snapple)* 100
raspberry *(Nestea)* 78
Tea, iced, mix:
lemon flavor *(Lipton),* 1⅔ tbsp. 90
w/out lemon *(Lipton),* 1⅔ tbsp. 80
Teff seed or flour *(Arrowhead Mills),* 2 oz. 200
Tempeh, ½ cup 165
Teriyaki entree, frozen, stir-fry *(Lean Cuisine),* 10 oz. . . . 290
Teriyaki sauce, 1 tbsp., except as noted:
(House of Tsang Korean Teriyaki) 30
(World Harbors Maui Mountain), 2 tbsp. 70
baste and glaze *(Kikkoman)* 50
baste and glaze, w/honey and pineapple *(Kikkoman)* 80
marinade *(Lawry's)* 20

marinade and *(Kikkoman/Kikkoman* Lite) 15
marinade and, roasted garlic *(Kikkoman)* 25
Polynesian *(Trader Vic's)* 15
Thai sauce *(World Harbors* Nong Khai Mountain),
   2 tbsp. 40
Thuringer cervelat, see "Summer sausage"
Thyme, ground, 1 tsp. 4
Thymus, 4 oz.:
beef, braised 362
veal, braised 197
Tilefish, meat only:
raw, 4 oz. 108
baked, broiled, or microwaved, 4 oz. 167
Tiramisu, see "Cake, frozen"
Toaster muffins and pastries, 1 piece:
all varieties *(Pop-Tarts* Low Fat) 190
apple cinnamon *(Pop-Tarts)* 210
berry, wild *(Toaster Strudel* Wildberry) 190
berry, wild, frosted *(Pop-Tarts)* 210
blueberry *(Natural Touch)* 180
blueberry, regular or frosted *(Pop-Tarts)* 200
brown sugar-cinnamon *(Pop-Tarts)* 210
cherry, regular or frosted *(Pop-Tarts)* 200
chocolate fudge or chocolate-vanilla *(Pop-Tarts)* 200
chocolate, milk, graham *(Pop-Tarts)* 210
date/walnut *(Natural Touch)* 200
grape, frosted *(Pop-Tarts)* 200
pizza, see "Pizza pockets"
strawberry, frosted *(Pop-Tarts)* 210
strawberry, regular or frosted *(Pop-Tarts)* 200
watermelon, wild, frosted *(Pop-Tarts)* 210
Tofu, fresh:
extra firm *(Nasoya),* 1/5 of 1-lb. block 90
firm *(Frieda's),* 3 oz. 60
firm *(Nasoya),* 1/5 of 1-lb. block 80
silken *(Nasoya),* 1/5 of 1-lb. block 50
soft *(Nasoya),* 1/6 of 1-lb. block 60
Tofu dishes, mix, dry:
burger *(Fantastic Foods),* 1/8 cup 70
chow mein, mandarin *(Fantastic Foods),* 5/8 cup 170

Tofu dishes, mix *(cont.)*
shells 'n curry *(Fantastic Foods)*, ½ cup 200
Stroganoff, creamy *(Fantastic Foods)*, ½ cup 190
Tom and Jerry, batter *(Trader Vic's)*, 1 tbsp. 116
Tomatillo:
(Frieda's), 3 oz. 25
(La Victoria Entero), 5 pieces, 4.5 oz. 40
crushed *(La Victoria)*, 4.5 oz. 45
Tomato:
raw, 2⅗″ tomato 26
raw, chopped, ½ cup 19
dried, see "Tomato, dried"
Tomato, canned, ½ cup, except as noted:
whole *(Del Monte)* 25
whole, peeled *(Progresso)* 25
whole, peeled *(Progresso* Italian Style) 20
whole, peeled, w/basil *(Muir Glen)* 30
chunky, chili style *(Del Monte)* 30
chunky, pasta style *(Del Monte)* 45
crushed *(Muir Glen)* 25
crushed *(Progresso)* 20
diced *(Del Monte/Del Monte* No Salt) 25
diced *(Muir Glen/Muir Glen* No Salt) 25
diced, w/basil, garlic, oregano *(Del Monte)* 50
diced, w/garlic or pepper and onion *(Del Monte)* 40
diced, w/garlic and onion *(Muir Glen)* 25
w/green chilies or jalapeños *(Old El Paso)*, ¼ cup 10
w/green chilies, diced *(Muir Glen)* 25
paste or puree, see "Tomato paste" and "Tomato
   puree"
stewed or wedges *(Del Monte)* 35
stewed, classic or Mexican *(Green Giant)* 35
stewed, Cajun or Mexican *(Del Monte)* 35
stewed, Italian *(Del Monte)* 30
stewed, Italian *(Green Giant)* 30
Tomato, dried:
1 piece (32 pieces per cup) 5
halves *(Sonoma)*, 2–3 pieces 15
in oil *(Christopher Ranch)*, 1 oz., approx. 6 pieces 80
Tomato, green, 2⅗″ tomato 30

Tomato, pickled *(Hebrew National/Shorr's)*, 1 oz. 4
Tomato, sun-dried, see "Tomato, dried"
Tomato appetizer, 1 oz.:
w/eggplant *(Sabra Matbucha Salad)* 18
w/vegetables *(Sabra Turkish Salad)* 13
Tomato dip, sun-dried *(Marie's)*, 2 tbsp. 140
Tomato juice, 8 fl. oz.:
(Campbell's/Campbell's Healthy Request/Low Sodium) 50
(Del Monte) 50
(Del Monte Not from Concentrate) 40
(Muir Glen From Organic Concentrate) 60
(Muir Glen From Concentrate) 40
(Sacramento) 35
Tomato paste *(Progresso)*, 2 tbsp. 30
Tomato preserve *(Smucker's)*, 1 tbsp. 50
Tomato puree, ¼ cup:
(Muir Glen) 20
(Progresso) 25
thick *(Progresso)* 20
Tomato sauce, canned (see also "Pasta sauce"), ¼
cup:
(Del Monte/Del Monte No Salt) 20
(Muir Glen Chunky/Organic/No Salt) 20
(Progresso) 20
Tomato-beef cocktail *(Beefamato)*, 8 fl. oz. 80
Tomato-chile cocktail *(Snap-E-Tom)*, 10 fl. oz. 60
Tomato-clam cocktail *(Clamato)*, 8 fl. oz. 100
Tongue, braised:
beef, 4 oz. 321
veal (calf), 4 oz. 229
Tortellini (see also "Tortelloni"), refrigerated:
cheese *(Contadina)*, ¾ cup 250
cheese *(Di Giorno)*, ¾ cup 260
cheese, w/red pepper, hot *(Di Giorno)*, 1 cup 310
cheese, three *(Contadina)*, ¾ cup 250
chicken and herb *(Contadina)*, ¾ cup 260
chicken and herb *(Di Giorno)*, 1 cup 260
w/meat *(Di Giorno)*, ¾ cup 290
mozzarella-garlic *(Di Giorno)*, 1 cup 300
mushroom *(Di Giorno)*, 1 cup 290

spinach cheese *(Contadina),* ¾ cup 260
Tortelloni (see also "Tortellini"), refrigerated, 1 cup:
cheese and herb *(Contadina)* 320
chicken and prosciutto *(Contadina)* 360
garlic and cheese *(Contadina* Light) 280
mushroom and cheese *(Contadina)* 290
tomato, sun-dried *(Contadina)* 320
Tortilla, 1 piece, except as noted:
corn, yellow or white *(Tyson),* 3 pieces, 1.9 oz. 140
flour *(Mesa* 6″) 80
flour *(Old El Paso/Old El Paso* Refrigerated) 130
flour *(Old El Paso* Refrigerated Low Fat) 110
flour *(Tyson),* 1.4 oz. 120
flour *(Tyson),* 1.9 oz. 170
flour, jalapeño-cilantro or sun-dried tomato *(Tumaro's*
 Burrito Size) 150
flour, whole wheat *(Tortilla),* 1.4 oz. 120
flour, heat pressed *(Tyson),* 2 pieces, 1.9 oz. 170
soft taco *(Old El Paso),* 2 pieces 160
soft taco *(Old El Paso* Refrigerated), 1 piece 110
Tortilla chips, see "Corn chips and similar snacks"
Trail mix:
(Eden Fruit & Nuts), 1 oz. 160
(Sonoma), ¼ cup 160
Trout (see also "Sea trout"), meat only, 4 oz.:
mixed species, raw 168
mixed species, baked, broiled, or microwaved 215
rainbow, farmed, raw 156
rainbow, farmed, baked, broiled, or microwaved 192
rainbow, wild, raw 135
rainbow, wild, baked, broiled, or microwaved 170
Trout, smoked, peppered *(Spence & Co.),* 2 oz. 100
Tuna, meat only, 4 oz.:
bluefin, raw 163
bluefin, baked, broiled, or microwaved 209
skipjack, raw 117
skipjack, baked, broiled, or microwaved 150
yellowfin, raw 123
yellowfin, baked, broiled, or microwaved 158

Tuna, canned, drained, 2 oz. or ¼ cup:

chunk light, in oil *(StarKist)* 110
chunk light or white, in water *(StarKist)* 60
solid, in olive oil *(Progresso)* 160
solid white, in oil *(StarKist)* 90
solid white, in water *(StarKist)* 70
"Tuna," vegetarian, canned *(Worthington Tuno)*,
   ⅓ cup 80
Tuna entree, frozen, noodle:
(Stouffer's Casserole), 10-oz. pkg. 320
chunky *(Marie Callender's)*, 12-oz. pkg. 960
grilled, barbecue *(Mrs. Paul's/Van de Kamp's)*, 1 fillet . . . 100
grilled, sesame teriyaki *(Mrs. Paul's/Van de Kamp's)*,
   1 fillet 110
Tuna entree mix, 1 cup*, except as noted:
au gratin *(Tuna Helper)* 300
broccoli, cheesy *(Tuna Helper)* 290
broccoli, creamy *(Tuna Helper)* 310
cheddar, garden *(Tuna Helper)* 290
fettuccine Alfredo *(Tuna Helper)* 310
pasta, cheesy *(Tuna Helper)* 280
pasta, creamy *(Tuna Helper)* 300
pasta salad *(Tuna Helper)*, ⅔ cup* 380
pot pie *(Tuna Helper)* 440
Romanoff *(Tuna Helper)* 280
tetrazzini or tuna melt *(Tuna Helper)* 300
Tuna salad, regular or chunky *(Wampler)*, ⅓ cup 180
Tuna spread *(Underwood)*, ¼ cup, 2 oz. 50
Turban squash *(Frieda's)*, ¾ cup, 3 oz. 30
Turbot, European, meat only:
raw, 4 oz. 108
baked, broiled, or microwaved, 4 oz. 138
Turkey, fresh, all classes, roasted:
meat, w/skin, 4 oz. 236
meat only, 4 oz. 193
meat only, diced, 1 cup 238
skin only, 1 oz. 125
dark meat, w/skin, 4 oz. 251
dark meat only, 4 oz. 212
light meat, w/skin, 4 oz. 223

Turkey *(cont.)*
light meat only, 4 oz. 178
breast, w/skin, ½ breast, 1.9 lb. (4.2 lbs. raw w/bone) . . .1637
ground, see "Turkey ground"
leg, w/skin, 1.2 lb. (1.5 lbs. raw w/bone) 1133
wing, w/skin:, 6.6 oz. (9.9 oz. raw w/bone) 426
Turkey, frozen or refrigerated, cooked:
whole, oven-roasted *(Shady Brook Farms)*, 2 oz. 90
breast *(Perdue* Whole or Half), 3 oz. 170
breast, honey roasted *(Shady Brook Farms)*, 2 oz. 60
breast, smoked *(Shady Brook Farms)*, 3 oz. 130
drumstick, smoked *(Shady Brook Farms)*, 3 oz. 180
meatballs, Italian *(Shady Brook Farms)*, 3 oz. 130
thigh *(Perdue)*, 3 oz. 180
wing, roasted *(Perdue* Drummettes), 3½-oz. piece 180
wing, smoked *(Shady Brook Farms)*, 3 oz. 200
Turkey, ground, raw, 4 oz.:
(Shady Brook Farms 85% Turkey) 220
(Wampler/Wampler Burger) 210
breast *(Shady Brook Farms)* 120
burger, barbecue *(Wampler)* 220
burger, specially seasoned *(Wampler)* 180
lean or burgers *(Shady Brook Farms)* 170
meatloaf *(Shady Brook Farms)* 150
"Turkey," vegetarian:
canned *(Worthington* Turkee), 3 slices 170
frozen, smoked, sliced *(Worthington)*, 3 slices 140
Turkey bacon *(Louis Rich)*, ½-oz. piece 35
Turkey bologna *(Wampler)*, 2 oz. 100
Turkey dinner, frozen, 1 pkg.:
breast *(Healthy Choice)* 280
and gravy, w/dressing *(Banquet)* 560
and gravy, w/dressing *(Marie Callender's)* 530
Turkey entree, frozen, 1 pkg., except as noted:
(Lean Cuisine Homestyle), 9⅜ oz. 230
breast *(Healthy Choice* Traditional), 10.5 oz. 290
breast, w/rice pilaf *(Marie Callender's)*, 11.75 oz. 320
chili, see "Chili entree,"
glazed tenderloins *(Lean Cuisine Cafe Classics)*, 9 oz. . . . 240
w/gravy, dressing *(Banquet Extra Helping)*, 17 oz. 630

w/gravy, dressing *(Marie Callender's)*, 14 oz. 500
pie *(Banquet)*, 7-oz. pie 370
pie *(Marie Callender's)*, 9.5 oz. 610
pie *(Stouffer's)*, 10-oz. pie 530
roast *(Healthy Choice* Country Inn), 10 oz. 250
roast *(Lean Cuisine Skillet Sensations)*, ½ of 24-oz.
   pkg. 220
roast *(Stouffer's* Homestyle), 9⅝ oz. 310
roast, breast *(Lean Cuisine American Favorites)*, 9¾ oz. . 270
roast, breast *(Lean Cuisine Hearty Portions)*, 14 oz. . . . 350
roast, breast *(Stouffer's Hearty Portions)*, 16 oz. 490
roast, honey, breast *(Banquet)*, 9 oz. 270
roast, w/mushrooms *(Healthy Choice* Country), 8.5 oz. . 220
sausage, w/peppers and onions *(Wampler)*, ⅑ pkg. 210
sliced, gravy and *(Banquet* Family), 2 slices w/gravy . . . 150
tetrazzini *(Stouffer's)*, 10 oz. 360
white meat, mostly *(Banquet* Meal), 9.25 oz. 280
Turkey frankfurter, see "Frankfurter"
Turkey giblets, simmered, diced, 1 cup 243
Turkey gravy, canned, ¼ cup:
(Franco-American) 25
(Franco-American Fat Free) 20
(Franco-American Slow Roasted) 30
Turkey ham, 2 oz.:
(Healthy Deli) 80
(Wampler) 50
Black Forest *(Shady Brook Farms)* 70
Black Forest or smoked *(Wampler)* 60
Turkey ham salad *(Wampler)*, ⅓ cup 150
Turkey liver, see "Liver"
Turkey lunch meat (see also "Turkey ham," etc.), 2 oz.
   breast, except as noted:
(Boar's Head Premium/*Ovengold/Salsalito)* 60
browned *(Healthy Choice)* 50
honey cured, Champagne glazed *(Black Bear)* 70
honey roasted *(Healthy Deli)* 60
honey roasted, w/cracked pepper *(Shady Brook Farms)* . . . 60
maple honey *(Boar's Head Maple Glazed Honey Coat)* 70
orange flavor *(Healthy Deli)* 65
oven roasted *(Black Bear)* 50

Turkey lunch meat *(cont.)*

oven roasted *(Boar's Head* Golden/Golden Skinless) 60
oven roasted *(Healthy Choice)* 45
oven roasted *(Healthy Deli* Gourmet) 60
oven roasted, glazed *(Healthy Deli* Gourmet) 60
oven roasted, Italian *(Healthy Deli)* 70
oven roasted, and white *(Healthy Choice),* 1-oz. slice 30
natural roasted *(Shady Brook Farms* Carved) 60
pan roasted *(Wampler)* 50
peppered *(Shady Brook Farms* Carved) 60
peppered *(Wampler)* 40
roasted *(Healthy Choice* Hearty Deli), 3 slices, 2 oz. 60
rotisserie *(Wampler)* 50
salsa *(Healthy Choice)* 60
slow-roasted, browned *(Shady Brook Farms)* 60
smoked *(Boar's Head Cracked Pepper Mill)* 60
smoked *(Healthy Deli)* 60
smoked, hickory *(Boar's Head)* 70
smoked, mesquite *(Healthy Deli)* 60
smoked, skinless *(Healthy Choice)* 50
smoked, white *(Oscar Mayer),* 1-oz. slice 30
Southwest grill *(Healthy Choice)* 60
spiced *(Wampler* Classic) 70
Tex-Mex *(Black Bear)* 60
Turkey pastrami, 2 oz.:
(Boar's Head) 60
(Healthy Deli) 70
(Wampler) 80
Turkey pocket, frozen, 4.5-oz. piece:
broccoli and cheese *(Lean Pockets)* 250
and ham, w/cheese *(Hot Pockets)* 300
and ham, w/cheese, cheddar *(Lean Pockets)* 270
and ham, w/cheese, Swiss *(Croissant Pockets)* 290
Turkey salami *(Wampler),* 2 oz. 90
Turkey sausage, see "Sausage"
Turmeric, ground, 1 tsp. 8
Turnip:
fresh, boiled, cubed, ½ cup 14
fresh, boiled, mashed, ½ cup 21
frozen, boiled, drained, 4 oz. 26

Turnip greens, 1/2 cup:
fresh, raw, chopped 7
fresh, boiled, chopped 15
canned *(Allens/Sunshine)* 25
canned, chopped, w/diced turnip *(Allens/Sunshine)* 30
frozen, w/diced turnip *(Seabrook)* 30
Turnover, refrigerated:
apple *(Pillsbury),* 2-oz. piece 170
cherry *(Pillsbury),* 2-oz. piece 180

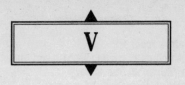

V

FOOD AND MEASURE   **CALORIES**

Veal, meat only, 4 oz.:
cubed, lean only, braised or stewed 213
ground, broiled 195
leg, roasted, lean w/fat 181
leg, roasted, lean only 170
loin, roasted, lean w/fat 246
loin, roasted, lean only 198
rib, roasted, lean w/fat 259
rib, roasted, lean only 201
shoulder, whole, braised, lean w/fat 259
shoulder, whole, braised, lean only 226
shoulder, whole, roasted, lean w/fat 209
shoulder, whole, roasted, lean only 193
sirloin, roasted, lean w/fat 229
sirloin, roasted, lean only 191
Veal entree, parmigiana, frozen:
(Banquet), 9 oz. 360
(Stouffer's Homestyle), 11⁷/₈ oz. 430
(Stouffer's Hearty Portions), 17¹/₂ oz. 630
patties *(Banquet* Family), 1 patty w/sauce 230
Vegetable burger, see "Burger, vegetarian"
Vegetable dip mix* garden *(Hidden Valley),* 2 tbsp. 70
Vegetable dip *(Heluva* Good), 2 tbsp. 60
Vegetable dishes, frozen (see also specific listings):
au gratin *(Cascadian Farm Veggie Bowl),* 9 oz. 170
pot pie *(Amy's),* 7.5 oz. 360
pot pie *(Amy's* Country), 7.5 oz. 370
pot pie *(Amy's* Nondairy), 7.5 oz. 320
pot pie, cheese *(Banquet),* 7 oz. 340
Vegetable entree, frozen, see "Vegetable dishes,
  frozen"
Vegetable entree, packaged, w/rice, 1 pkg.:
creamy, w/pistachos/raisins *(Tamarind Tree* Navratan
  Korma) 430

Vegetable entree *(cont.)*
peas and mushrooms *(Tamarind Tree Dhingri Mutter)* . . . 290
spicy garden *(Tamarind Tree Jalfrazi)* 310
Vegetable juice, 8 fl. oz., except as noted:
(Dole), 12 fl. oz. 90
(Muir Glen/Muir Glen Reduced Sodium/Spicy) 70
(V8 Low Sodium/Lightly Tangy) 60
(V8/V8 Healthy Request Picante/Spicy) 50
spicy blend *(Dole),* 12 fl. oz. 80
Vegetable pie, see "Vegetable dishes, frozen"
Vegetable pocket, frozen, 1 piece:
Bar-B-Q *(Ken & Robert's Veggie Pockets)* 290
Greek or Oriental *(Ken & Robert's Veggie Pockets)* . . . 250
Indian *(Ken & Robert's Veggie Pockets)* 260
Mediterranean or roasted vegetables *(Amy's)* 220
pot pie *(Amy's)* 230
Santa Fe or pot pie *(Ken & Robert's Veggie Pockets)* . . 250
Tex-Mex *(Ken & Robert's Veggie Pockets)* 280
Vegetables, see specific listings
Vegetables, mixed, canned, ½ cup, except as noted:
(Del Monte/Del Monte No Salt) 40
(Green Giant) 60
(Green Giant Garden Medley) 40
(Seneca/Seneca No Salt/Stew) 45
Vegetables, mixed, frozen (see also "Vegetable dishes,
    frozen"), ¾ cup, except as noted:
(Green Giant) 50
(Green Giant Harvest Fresh), ⅔ cup 50
(Seneca), ⅔ cup 60
Alfredo *(Green Giant)* 80
in butter sauce *(Green Giant)* 70
California *(Cascadian Farm),* ⅔ cup 20
in cheese sauce *(Cascadian Farm Medley),* ⅔ cup 80
Chinese stir-fry *(Cascadian Farm),* 1 cup 25
gardener's blend *(Cascadian Farm)* 57
Italian *(Seneca)* 30
Oriental, blend or stir-fry *(Seneca)* 25
Santa Fe blend *(Cascadian Farm)* 60
Scandinavian blend or soup mix *(Seneca)* 40
stew, hearty *(Cascadian Farm),* ⅔ cup 45

teriyaki *(Green Giant)*, 1¼ cup 100
Thai stir-fry *(Cascadian Farm)* 25
winter blend *(Seneca)* 25
Vegetarian dishes (see also "Vegetarian entree" and
  specific listings):
canned *(Loma Linda Swiss Stake)*, 1 piece 120
canned *(Worthington Numete/Protose)*, ⅜" slice 130
canned, choplet *(Worthington)*, 2 pieces 90
canned, cuts, dinner *(Loma Linda)*, 2 pieces 90
canned, cutlet *(Worthington)*, 1 piece 70
frozen *(Worthington FriPats)*, 1 patty 130
frozen *(Worthington Stakelets)*, 1 piece 140
frozen, croquettes *(Worthington* Golden), 4 pieces 210
frozen, roast, dinner *(Worthington)*, ¾" slice 180
Vegetarian entree, frozen (see also specific listings):
Aztec or Cajun *(Cascadian Farm Meals for a Small
  Planet)*, ½ bag 230
Indian *(Cascadian Farm Meals for a Small Planet)*,
  ½ bag 250
Mediterranean *(Cascadian Farm Meals for a Small
  Planet)*, ½ bag 215
mu shu *(Fantastic Wrap Stuffers)*, 16 oz. 220
Oriental *(Cascadian Farm Meals for a Small Planet)*,
  ½ bag 260
pot pie, see "Vegetable dishes, frozen"
Santa Fe *(Fantastic Wrap Stuffers)*, 16 oz. 240
shepherd's pie *(Amy's* Nondairy), 8 oz. 160
Spanish *(Fantastic Wrap Stuffers)*, 16 oz. 220
teriyaki *(Fantastic Wrap Stuffers)*, 16 oz. 230
Vegetarian foods, see specific listings
Venison, meat only, roasted, 4 oz. 179
Vienna sausage, canned:
(Libby's/Libby's BBQ), 3 links 130
chicken *(Libby's)*, 3 links 100
Vine spinach, raw, untrimmed, 1 lb. 86
Vinegar, 1 tbsp.:
all varieties, except balsamic *(Progresso)* 0
balsamic *(Progresso)* 10

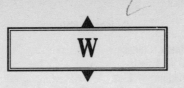

W

FOOD AND MEASURE   **CALORIES**

Waffle, frozen, 2 pieces, except as noted:
(Aunt Jemima Homestyle) 200
(Aunt Jemima Lowfat) 160
(Belgian Chef), 2.6 oz. 180
(Eggo Homestyle) 220
(Eggo Homestyle Low Fat) 180
(Eggo Minis Homestyle), 3 sets of 4 pieces 260
(Eggo Nutri-Grain) 190
(Eggo Nutri-Grain Low Fat) 160
(Eggo Special K) 120
(Hungry Jack Homestyle) 180
(Hungry Jack Homestyle Low Fat) 170
apple cinnamon *(Eggo)* 220
apple cinnamon *(Hungry Jack)* 200
blueberry *(Aunt Jemima)* 210
blueberry *(Hungry Jack)* 210
blueberry, buttermilk, or strawberry *(Eggo)* 220
buttermilk *(Aunt Jemima)* 200
buttermilk *(Hungry Jack)* 180
cinnamon toast *(Eggo)*, 3 sets of 4 pieces 290
multibran *(Eggo Nutri-Grain)* 180
multigrain *(Hungry Jack)* 180
nut and honey *(Eggo)* 240
oat, golden *(Eggo)* 150
raisin and bran *(Eggo Nutri-Grain)* 210
wildberry *(Hungry Jack)* 200
Waffle mix, see "Pancake mix"
Walnut, dried:
(Paradise/Wild Swan), ¼ cup, 1 oz. 190
black, shelled, 1 oz. 172
English or Persian, shelled, 1 oz. 182
English or Persian, halves, 1 cup 642
Walnut topping, in syrup *(Smucker's)*, 2 tbsp. 170

Water chestnuts, Chinese:

fresh *(Frieda's)*, 1 tbsp. 30

canned, 4 medium or 1 oz. 14

canned, sliced *(Sun Luck)*, ¼ cup 15

Water spinach, see "Spinach, water"

Watercress:

10 sprigs, 11¼" 3

chopped, ½ cup 2

Watermelon:

1" slice, 10" diam. 152

diced, ½ cup 25

Watermelon, yellow, seedless *(Frieda's)*, 2 cups,

9.9 oz. 90

Watermelon juice *(After the Fall)*, 8 fl. oz. 90

Watermelon seed, dried, 1 oz. 158

Wax beans:

fresh, see "Green bean"

canned, cut *(Del Monte/Del Monte* Golden), ½ cup 20

canned, cut *(Seneca/Seneca* No Salt), ½ cup 25

frozen *(Seabrook)*, ⅔ cup 25

Welsh rarebit, frozen *(Stouffer's* Side Dish), ¼ cup 110

Wendy's, 1 serving:

sandwiches:

    bacon cheeseburger, Jr. 380

    Big Bacon Classic 580

    cheeseburger Jr. 320

    cheeseburger Jr, deluxe 360

    cheeseburger Kid's Meal 320

    chicken, grilled 310

    chicken, breaded 440

    chicken, spicy 410

    chicken club 470

    hamburger, single, plain 360

    hamburger, single, w/everything 420

    hamburger Jr. 270

    hamburger Kid's Meal 270

*Fresh Stuffed Pitas,*w/dressing:

    chicken Caesar 490

    classic Greek 440

    garden ranch chicken 480

garden veggie 400
pita dressing, Caesar vinaigrette 70
pita dressing, garden ranch sauce 50
chicken nuggets, 5 pieces 230
nuggets sauce, 1 pkt.:
  barbecue 45
  honey mustard 130
  sweet and sour 50
chili:
  small, 8 oz. 210
  large, 12 oz. 310
  cheddar cheese, shredded, 2 tbsp. 70
  saltine crackers, 2 pieces 25
baked potato:
  plain, 10 oz. 310
  bacon and cheese 530
  broccoli and cheese 470
  cheese 570
  chili and cheese 630
  sour cream and chive 380
  sour cream or whipped margarine pkt. 60
french fries:
  small 270
  medium 390
  Biggie 470
  Great Biggie 570
salads-to-go, fresh, w/out dressing:
  Caesar side salad or deluxe garden 110
  grilled chicken 200
  side salad 60
  taco salad 380
  taco chips, 15 pieces 100
  soft breadstick, 1 piece 130
dressing, 2 tbsp., except as noted:
  blue cheese 180
  French 120
  French, fat free 35
  Italian, reduced fat/calorie 40
  Italian Caesar 150
  ranch, *Hidden Valley* 100

Wendy's,* dressing *(cont.)
ranch, *Hidden Valley,* reduced fat/cal. 60
salad oil, 1 tbsp. 120
Thousand Islands 90
wine vinegar, 1 tbsp. 0
desserts:
chocolate chip cookie 270
Frosty, small 330
Frosty, medium 440
Frosty, large 540
Wheat, whole-grain, durum, 1 cup 650
Wheat, parboiled, see "Bulgur"
Wheat bran (see also "Cereal"), ¼ cup, except as noted:
(Arrowhead Mills) 35
crude, 2 tbsp. 15
toasted *(Kretschmer)* 30
Wheat flakes *(Arrowhead Mills),* ⅓ cup 110
Wheat flour, ¼ cup, except as noted:
all-purpose, white *(Gold Medal/Gold Medal* Organic) 100
all purpose, white *(Pillsbury)* 100
bread *(Gold Medal/Red Band* Better for Bread) 100
bread, wheat *(Gold Medal* Better for Bread) 110
bread, white *(Pillsbury)* 100
cake, white *(Betty Crocker Softasilk)* 100
cake, white *(Swan's Down)* 100
gluten *(Arrowhead Mills),* 3 tbsp. 35
gluten *(General Mills* Supreme Hygluten) 100
pastry *(Arrowhead Mills)* 110
presifted *(Pillsbury* Shake & Blend) 100
presifted *(Wondra)* 100
self-rising, white *(Gold Medal/Robin Hood)* 100
self-rising, white *(Pillsbury)* 100
self-rising, white, unbleached *(Gold Medal/Robin Hood)* . . 100
whole wheat *(Pillsbury)* 120
whole wheat, stone ground *(Arrowhead Mills)* 130
Wheat germ *(Kretschmer),* 2 tbsp. 50
Whelk, meat only, raw, 4 oz. 156
Whipped topping, see "Cream topping"

White Castle, 1 serving:
sandwiches:
    breakfast 340
    cheeseburger 160
    cheeseburger, bacon 200
    cheeseburger, double 285
    chicken ring 170
    fish 160
    hamburger 135
    hamburger, double 235
chicken rings, 6 pieces 310
sides:
    cheese sticks, 5 pieces 491
    fries, small 115
    onion rings, 8 pieces 460
shakes, chocolate, 14 oz. 220
shakes, vanilla, 14 oz. 230
White bean, ½ cup:
dried, boiled 125
dried, small, boiled 127
canned, w/liquid 153
Whitefish, meat only:
raw, 4 oz. 153
baked, broiled, or microwaved, 4 oz. 195
smoked, 4 oz. 122
Whiting, meat only:
raw, 4 oz. 102
baked, broiled, or microwaved, 4 oz. 130
Wiener, see "Frankfurter"
Wild rice:
raw *(Fantastic Foods),* ¼ cup 140
raw *(Frieda's),* ¼ cup 120
cooked, 1 cup 166
Wild rice dishes, see "Rice dishes"
Wine, 1 fl. oz.:
dessert or apertif[1] 41

---

[1] *Includes fortified wines containing more than 15% alcohol, such as port, sherry, vermouth, etc.*

dry or table[1] 25
Wine cooler, apple
(Bartles & Jaymes), 12-oz. bottle:
berry 220
berry, Brazilian mist 210
Fuzzy navel or Oriental dragon fruit 250
kiwi strawberry or strawberry daiquiri 230
Margarita 270
original 200
tropical 240
Winged bean, ½ cup:
fresh, raw, sliced 11
fresh, boiled, drained 12
dried, boiled 126
Wolf fish, Atlantic, meat only:
raw, 4 oz. 109
baked, broiled, or microwaved, 4 oz. 139
Wonton wrapper:
(Frieda's), 4 pieces 80
(Nasoya), 5 pieces 90
Worcestershire sauce, 1 tsp.:
(Crosse & Blackwell) 5
(Lea & Perrins) 5
(French's) 0
white wine *(Lea & Perrins)* 0

[1] *Includes wines containing less than 15% alcohol, such as burgundy, Chablis, champagne, etc.*

Y–Z

Yam, ½ cup:
baked or boiled 79
canned or frozen, see "Sweet potato"
Yam, mountain, Hawaiian, steamed, cubed, ½ cup 59
Yam bean tuber:
raw *(Frieda's* Jicama), ¾ cup, 3 oz. 35
boiled, drained, 4 oz. 43
Yard-long bean:
fresh, raw, sliced, ½ cup 22
fresh, boiled, drained, sliced, ½ cup 25
dried, boiled, ½ cup 102
Yeast, baker's, all varieties *(Fleischmann's)*, ¼ tsp. 0
Yellow beans, dried, boiled, ½ cup 126
Yellow squash, see "Crookneck squash"
Yellowtail, meat only:
raw, 4 oz. 166
baked, broiled, or microwaved, 4 oz. 212
Yogurt, 8 oz., except as noted:
plain *(Breyers* 1.5% Milkfat) 130
plain *(Columbo* Fat Free) 110
plain *(Dannon* Fat Free) 110
plain *(Dannon* Lowfat/Organic) 150
plain *(Friendship)* 150
all flavors *(Columbo* Light) 100
all flavors *(Dannon* Light) 100
all flavors *(Yoplait* Custard Style), 6 oz. 190
all fruit flavors *(Dannon* Chunky Fruit), 6 oz. 160
all fruit flavors *(Dannon* Fruit on the Bottom) 240
all fruit flavors *(Yoplait)*, 6 oz. 180
all fruit flavors *(Yoplait* Light), 6 oz. 90
all fruit flavors *(Yoplait* 99% Fat Free), 4 oz. 120
all fruit flavors *(Yoplait* Trix), 6 oz. 190
all fruit flavors, except banana/strawberry *(Columbo* Fat
    Free) 200

Yogurt *(cont.)*

banana/strawberry *(Columbo Fat Free)* 220
berries, mixed *(Breyers 1% Milkfat)* 250
blueberry *(Breyers 1% Milkfat)* 250
blueberry *(Light n' Lively 1% Milkfat), 4.4 oz.* 140
café au lait *(Yoplait), 6 oz.* 170
cappuccino *(Columbo Fat Free)* 170
cheesecake *(Dannon Double Delights), 6 oz.* 170
cherry, black *(Breyers 1% Milkfat)* 260
cherry vanilla *(Dannon Chunky Fruit), 6 oz.* 160
cherry vanilla *(Dannon Sprinkl'ins), 4.1 oz.* 130
chocolate cheesecake *(Dannon Double Delights), 6 oz.* . . . 220
coconut cream pie *(Yoplait), 6 oz.* 200
coffee *(Breyers 1.5% Milkfat)* 220
coffee, cranberry-raspberry, or vanilla *(Dannon)* 210
French roast or lemon *(Columbo Fat Free)* 170
lemon *(Dannon)* 210
lemon, creamy *(Breyers 1.5% Milkfat)* 220
lemon meringue pie *(Dannon Double Delights), 6 oz.* . . . 180
peach *(Breyers 1% Milkfat)* 250
peach *(Light n' Lively 1% Milkfat), 4.4 oz.* 140
pineapple *(Breyers 1% Milkfat)* 250
pineapple *(Light n' Lively 1% Milkfat), 4.4 oz.* 140
raspberry *(Dannon Blended), 6 oz.* 110
raspberry, red *(Light n' Lively 1% Milkfat), 4.4 oz.* 130
raspberry or strawberry *(Breyers 1% Milkfat)* 250
strawberry *(Dannon Blended), 4 oz.* 110
strawberry *(Dannon Sprinkl'ins), 4.1 oz.* 130
strawberry *(Light n' Lively 1% Milkfat), 4.4 oz.* 140
strawberry banana *(Breyers 1% Milkfat)* 250
strawberry banana *(Dannon Blended), 4 oz.* 110
vanilla *(Breyers 1.5% Milkfat)* 220
vanilla *(Columbo Fat Free)* 170
vanilla, French *(Yoplait), 6 oz.* 180
vanilla caramel sundae *(Columbo Fat Free)* 220
Yogurt, frozen, ½ cup:
all flavors *(Dannon Fat Free)* 100
all flavors, except cookies and cream and chocolate
    fudge, German *(Columbo Nonfat)* 100
all fruit flavors *(Columbo Slender Sensations)* 60

banana split *(Blue Bell* Nonfat) 110
(Ben & Jerry's Cherry Garcia) 170
(Ben & Jerry's Chocolate Cherry Garcia) 190
caramel praline crunch *(Edy's/Dreyer's* Fat Free) 100
cherry, black, vanilla swirl *(Edy's/Dreyer's* Fat Free) 80
cherry chocolate chunk *(Edy's/Dreyer's)* 110
cherry vanilla *(Häagen-Dazs)* 140
chocolate *(Breyers)* 130
chocolate *(Columbo* Slender Sensations) 70
chocolate *(Dannon* Lowfat) 120
chocolate *(Häagen-Dazs)* 140
chocolate, Old World *(Columbo* Lowfat) 110
chocolate brownie chunk *(Edy's/Dreyer's)* 120
chocolate chip cookie dough *(Ben & Jerry's)* 200
chocolate fudge *(Edy's/Dreyer's* Fat Free) 100
chocolate fudge brownie *(Ben & Jerry's)* 190
chocolate fudge, German *(Columbo* Nonfat) 110
chocolate silk mousse *(Edy's/Dreyer's* Fat Free) 90
coffee *(Häagen-Dazs)* 140
coffee fudge sundae *(Edy's/Dreyer's* Fat Free) 100
cookie dough *(Edy's/Dreyer's)* 130
cookies and cream *(Columbo* Nonfat) 120
cookies and cream *(Edy's/Dreyer's)* 110
cookies in cream *(Breyers* Fat Free) 110
marble fudge *(Edy's/Dreyer's* Fat Free) 100
peach raspberry trifle *(Ben & Jerry's)* 180
peanut butter *(Columbo* Lowfat) 120
peanut butter *(Dannon* Lowfat) 120
strawberry *(Blue Bell* Nonfat) 120
strawberry *(Breyers* Fat Free) 100
strawberry *(Columbo* Lowfat) 110
strawberry cheesecake *(Blue Bell* Lowfat) 130
toffee crunch *(Edy's/Dreyer's Heath)* 120
toffee crunch, vanilla *(Ben & Jerry's Vanilla Heath)* 210
vanilla *(Blue Bell* Country Lowfat) 120
vanilla *(Breyers)* 120
vanilla *(Breyers* Fat Free) 100
vanilla *(Columbo* Slender Sensations) 60
vanilla *(Dannon* Fat Free Light) 70
vanilla *(Dannon* Lowfat) 110

Yogurt, frozen *(cont.)*
vanilla *(Edy's/Dreyer's)* 100
vanilla *(Edy's/Dreyer's* Fat Free) 80
vanilla *(Häagen-Dazs)* 140
vanilla, French or simply *(Columbo* Lowfat) 110
vanilla. bean *(Blue Bell* Nonfat) 110
vanilla chocolate *(Breyers* Fat Free Take Two) 100
vanilla swirl *(Edy's/Dreyer's* Fat Free) 80
vanilla chocolate strawberry *(Breyers)* 120
vanilla fudge *(Häagen-Dazs)* 160
vanilla fudge twirl *(Breyers* Fat Free) 110
vanilla raspberry swirl *(Häagen-Dazs)* 130
Yogurt bar, frozen, 1 bar:
all flavors *(Starburst)* 70
banana and strawberry *(Häagen-Dazs)* 90
cherry chocolate chip *(Ben & Jerry's Cherry Garcia)* . . . 260
chocolate and cherry *(Häagen-Dazs)* 100
chocolate and vanilla *(Häagen-Dazs)* 90
chocolate fudge *(Edy's)* 240
raspberry and vanilla *(Häagen-Dazs)* 90
Strawberry Cheesecake Craze (Häagen-Dazs Extras) . . . 220
strawberry daiquiri *(Häagen-Dazs)* 90
toffee crunch *(Edy's)* 250
Tropical Orange Passion (Häagen-Dazs) 100
vanilla almond *(Edy's)* 230
Yow choy sum *(Frieda's)*, 1 cup, 3 oz. 20
Yuca root *(Frieda's)*, 3 oz. 100
Zucchini:
fresh, raw, baby, 1 large, 3⅛" 3
fresh, boiled, drained, sliced, ½ cup 14
canned, Italian style *(Del Monte)*, ½ cup 30
canned, Italian style *(Progresso)*, ½ cup 50
frozen *(Seneca)*, ⅔ cup 15
Zucchini, breaded, frozen *(Empire)*, 1 piece 100
Zucchini, marinated, sun-dried, in jars *(Antica Italia)*,
   1 oz. 160